For Daniya
David Siroospour

Spinal Surgery Myths

A Surgeon's Personal Experience with Back Surgery

Dr. David Siroospour, MD FACS

Kennedy Gulch Press

Spinal Surgery Myths:
A Surgeon's Personal Experience with Back Surgery

Published by Kennedy Gulch Press

For further information:
Arbor Books
19 Spear Rd. Suite 301
Ramsey, NJ 07446
www.arborbooks.com

Printed in the United States of America

Spinal Surgery Myths:
A Surgeon's Personal Experience with Back Surgery
Dr. David Siroospour, MD FACS

1. Title 2. Author 3. Alternative Medicine

Library of Congress Control Number: 2009900909

ISBN-10: 0-9823362-0-9
ISBN-13: 978-0-9823362-0-5

Table of Contents

introduction

It has been a severe and relentless pursuit to rid my body of the intense, chronic pain I developed after two major spine surgeries. This chronic pain was much different than the manageable pain I had endured before my surgery. It was the kind of pain that exhausted my entire body. It started with my lower back and eventually moved its way down into my legs. The two spinal surgeries, one in the neck and one in the back, did not solve my exasperation—but rather added further problems to my health history.

When my injury occurred, I felt as if I were the only

one who had had a failed back surgery. And in the subsequent five years after my surgery, I traveled from pain clinic to pain clinic, from institute to institute, and considered that perhaps chronic pain was the "norm" after a major spine surgery. There were hundreds of people with the same condition and I eventually learned that my chronic pain was something that spine surgeons called "failed back syndrome."

"Failed back syndrome" is interesting nomenclature, don't you think? Perhaps, instead, we should call it "failed diagnosis syndrome."

I, myself, was a general surgeon at one time. I practiced from 1976 to 1988, after seven intricate years of surgical training. I was a solo practitioner in a small Iowa community, serving a large population of patients with varied health problems. I considered these patients parts of my family. And when they got sick, I lived with them day and night until they were well. My work—these people—were the most important thing in my life, only second to my own family.

I was trained much like a typical Western medicine

physician is trained today. I studied and looked at the human body as if it were a complex machine. And through surgery, I could fix the machine if something malfunctioned. I never believed in this thing called the "mind-body interaction" and I certainly did not believe in alternative medicine. To me, it was foolish. If treatment options weren't written in medical textbooks or in some prestigious medical journal, I did not believe they could be effective. End of story.

I harbored the idea that highly trained physicians, myself included, could fix and treat anything that came our way. My thinking was, if we couldn't fix the problem, then it must have been the patient's fault. Oftentimes, doctors believe the "illness" is all in the patient's head. Certainly it was *never* the fault of the brilliant medical system.

I had no idea—or maybe I just ignored the fact—that there were millions of people with chronic illness in this country who were desperately looking for help. But more importantly, I had no idea that these millions of people were usually unable to find any doctors to listen to them. If the lab tests were normal and the x-rays showed nothing, then how could the patient possibly be sick?

Then, one day, it was my turn. I got sick. More specifically, I developed a problem with my legs, so walking was difficult and awkward. I saw several specialists, which lead to several MRIs, CAT scans, EMGs and other extensive lab tests. The MRI results showed that I had spinal stenosis and deformities in my spine. My treating physician and I took this prognosis very seriously and knew that surgery was the best answer. Because I believed that Western medicine could diagnose and treat anything, I went through a horrendous, fourteen-hour surgery that basically ruined my life.

In the beginning, I thought I just had bad luck. After all, I knew failure could occasionally happen after any kind of surgery, but I guess you don't realize the severity of the situation until it bites you. Consequently, I had a huge awakening. I had to rethink everything I knew about medicine and the way I had been trained to think about it. Had my spine surgery been done for the wrong diagnosis? Perhaps it had been. Had the x-rays been correct? Yes, they probably had been. But still, nothing seemed to add up.

During my ruthless suffering, and after a countless number of failed treatments, I became extremely concerned with the validity of Western medicine. I felt as though it wouldn't be long before doctors realized that their way of practicing medicine was the cause of much patient agony after barbaric types of surgery.

Fortunately, it does not have to be this way any

longer. In order to treat patients correctly, doctors must first evaluate both the patients' minds and bodies, and study their health histories. There should be no separation between the mind and body. But because of their Western medicine training, doctors are not always taught to do that. "There's just not enough time."

Many physicians ignore patients as individuals. Instead of treating the patients, we tend to only treat their charts. We rely on x-ray and MRI findings to come up with diagnoses and coinciding treatments. Doctors do not spend enough time with each patient in the office. And in turn, the patients' visits are largely influenced by the quality of medical records and the impact of insurance companies.

My experience with back surgery is very common. Failed back surgeries and chronic pain are extremely high in American society. Statistics show that of the 200,000 back surgeries performed each year, twenty to forty percent result in various degrees of failed back surgery syndrome. It's now time to change the thought pattern about the diagnosis and treatment of chronic back pain.

It is my hope that you will learn from my mistakes and see the positive things that came out of my own ordeal. There have been tremendous success stories about using methods other than surgery and prescription drugs.

It is important that both the doctors and the patients learn to question the common diagnosis of back pain based on ordinary imaging techniques. MRIs, CAT scans and myleograms do not tell the whole story about a patient. They only show the image of his or her back at that moment.

It is time doctors tried other noninvasive, alternative treatments before resorting to the low success rate of spine surgery. Before any life-changing is analysis is made, we must understand the important interaction between the mind and the body, and the way it affects our physical, mental and emotional states of wellbeing. This crucial information will allow you to make informed decisions about your physical condition.

Patients need to take their health into their own hands if they are not getting results. They must actively participate in their own healing. Humans have an enormous capacity for healing, but this has to be recognized and explored before we can heal correctly. This book will start you along that path. Be well!

one

Considering Surgery—The Pain That Leads You There

The Mystery Pain

For most of us, it all starts with a mysterious pain that doesn't go away. We get a pain somewhere—oftentimes without knowing where it came from—that is debilitating enough to send us to the doctor for a checkup. Even though I am a doctor myself, I am no different than anyone in this regard.

It was a typical day for me. I was performing a fairly involved surgery on a patient. I was removing the thyroid gland—the gland in the front of the neck—of this young woman who had cancer. It was a delicate and meticulous surgery in which I had to pay attention to numerous anatomical structures. Things were progressing well. The area that I was operating on was free from oozing blood and I was able to identify and delineate most of the important structures.

Then, suddenly, in the midst of my work, I had a painful spasm in the muscles of my right hand. It was a spasm in my metacarpal bones, between my fingers and my wrist. These are the internal muscles of the hands. Essentially, it gave me a claw hand in the middle of this delicate surgery.

I turned around and immersed my hands in a hot basin of water, next to the operating table, to relieve the spasms. It helped temporarily, but the spasms returned after a few minutes of work. The nurses knew I often had problems with my hands. Most times, spasms will occur in a surgeon's hands after long procedures. I tried to shift the workload to my left hand and after a while, the same thing happened.

Spasms can be the most disturbing thing for a surgeon, who can be compared to a piano player in the middle of a concert. I was hoping that it was just fatigue in my hands from doing several surgeries a day. In the past, I'd had some hand spasms, but it had never been severe enough to affect my functioning during surgery. This time, it was quite severe, and it worried me.

If there was one thing I needed, it was to have steady hands. I decided to ask a colleague to scrub in with me for the rest of my operations that day because I was nervous that I wouldn't be able to finish the surgeries alone.

A few days later, I was performing a major colon cancer surgery in which I had to remove the entire rectum and do a colostomy. This surgery is literally like running a marathon for the muscles of the hands. I was in the middle of the second stage of that operation when the spasms came back. But this time, I was prepared, and I let my partner finish the surgery.

I consulted my physician. He ordered an EMG, which ruled out carpal tunnel syndrome. This test is used to detect neuromuscular abnormalities. When the test came back negative for carpal tunnel, it meant that there was no compression of the median or ulnar nerve at the wrist. These are the nerves that can get trapped and compressed by a tight band of tissue at the wrist, choking the underlying nerve and causing symptoms of carpal tunnel syndrome.

I consulted a neurologist, who ordered an MRI of my neck to rule out nerve entrapment or neck compression as the cause of my symptoms. When I received the results, my MRI made me very concerned. I had spinal stenosis at several levels in my neck.

Spinal stenosis is a narrowing of the spinal canal where the spinal cord passes through, putting it and the surrounding nerves under pressure. According to text books, spinal stenosis can cause numbness and pain in your extremities—legs, arms and shoulders. Sometimes, spinal stenosis in the neck can cause clumsiness of the hands, but I didn't have this symptom. It was the spasms that were the problem.

Even though the MRI showed degenerative disease in the spines of my neck, I did not have any pain in my neck at that time. I had always been very physically active, playing racquetball and tennis and lifting weights. Looking at the MRI, my neurologist suggested that I see a spine surgeon and prohibited me from doing any sport activities.

I looked at the MRI in shock. It looked so abnormal compared to the MRIs I was used to seeing in my practice. I never realized that most of the MRIs that I saw were of younger people with no major abnormalities. The neurologist assured me that my stenosis was the cause of my muscle spasms.

The psychological impact of this abnormal MRI finding was tremendous. I quit all physical activity and allowed myself to be disabled because my MRI was telling me that with that sort of picture, I *should* be disabled. I began having severe discomfort and spasms in my neck that I had not had before. Unfortunately, this is not unusual when patients are told that their spine is degenerating. The impact of knowing they have such degeneration is devastating and makes them act out the abnormality in their MRI.

In her famous book *Anatomy of the Spirit*, Dr. Caroline Myss wrote, "Our biography becomes our biology." She believes that the mind and the way that we think have an amazing influence on what we feel physically. Dr. Herbert Benson demonstrated something similar in his book, *Timeless Healing: The Power and Biology of Belief.* He noted that stress directly influences our health. And in her landmark work, *Molecules of Emotions*, Candace Pert elegantly and scientifically demonstrated how our emotions affect our physical health. She explained how our feelings, emotions and bodies are connected. "Through our mind," she said, "we can begin to understand how our body works." These feelings and issues seemed to all be happening to me at once.

The next thing I knew, I was sitting in front of a famous spine surgeon who had an incredible reputation and extensive training. He agreed with the diagnosis that the spasms were probably the result of spinal stenosis, but he thought my symptoms were somewhat atypical. He noted that when I bent my neck to perform surgeries, it constricted the artery in front of the spinal cord, called the anterior spinal artery, which further deprived the blood supply to the spinal cord, causing the spasm. Anatomically, that made perfect sense to me because I was a surgeon and a Western-trained physician.

His words still echoed in my head as I left his office: *"Your spinal cord is compressed like a pancake."* Surgery would be necessary. He told me that the goal of the surgery was to relieve pressure on the spinal cord and the spinal nerve by widening the spinal canal. This would be done by removing, trimming or realigning the involved parts contributing to the pressure. Usually, after removing that much bone from the vertebrae, they would have to fuse that segment of the spine. In my case, they had to fuse four levels in my neck.

Spinal fusion is a major surgical procedure that mingles and amalgamates joints together between the spine. As a result, the area that has been fused becomes much like a solid piece of bone, incapable of motion. The fusion process is done by placing pieces of bone graft between the spines. Either cadaver bone or the patient's can be used for grafting. After the fusion is completed, the area has to be immobilized so that the bones can heal correctly. This immobilization is done by an internal fixation using plates, screws and rods.

My physician assured me that he had done many spinal fusion surgeries, but there were still risks of paralysis and nerve injuries. The surgeon made me realize that it would be a major surgery with potential complications and a long recovery period. In other words, no walk in the park.

When I came out of the office, I was in pain. Spasms were moving through my neck, and there was some heaviness in my arms. I would have never known about my neck if I had not had the spasm in my hand.

In addition to the MRI of my neck, I decided to have an MRI on my back. I'd noticed some curvature in my back that was not yet painful, but it had worried me. In recent years, it had become more prominent. The curve of my back was not noticeable to other people but I was acutely aware of it. The MRI of my lower and mid-back showed that I also had spinal stenosis involving the lumbar vertebrae from L1 to L3.

Since childhood, I'd had spondylolisthesis, an abnormality wherein the lumbar vertebra has moved out of alignment with the one below it. It can move either forward or backward, and in my case it was a mild forward movement. My entire lumbar spine also had a front-to-back curvature called kyphosis that I'd developed over the years, but it was not painful. So, in addition to the neck abnormalities, I discovered that I had these back abnormalities as well.

Goodbye to My Career

At this time, I was at the peak of my surgical practice. I was fifty-nine and still had a few more years of my surgical career in front of me. But now, I was at a crossroads. I had to accept either that I would have little use of my hands for the rest of my life or that I had to go through a major surgery with no promise of success.

After a long, agonizing examination of my life, I chose to quit my practice and not have the surgery. It was the most traumatic time of my life. It was a painful retirement for me because I absolutely loved my profession. I was good at it. And I had an enormous practice with many patients whom I adored. Helping the people whom I considered family defined who I was as a person. All of my identity came from being a good doctor and a prudent, skilled surgeon. I felt I was losing who I was in this life.

At the same time, I had difficulties forgetting that my spine was compressed in my neck. The spasms in my hands continued despite my not using them as much. In fact, they got worse. It led me to finally give in and have the surgery two years later.

I went to a major university where the top spine surgeon still believed that the spasms were caused by spinal stenosis. This surgery was to take three to four hours. I felt like I had no other choice but to have the surgery and hope that it would fix the spasms in my hands and neck for good.

It took six months to recover from the trauma of this surgery and in the end, it did nothing to relieve the spasms in my hands. My initial impression as a physician was that my spinal cord was already damaged, and that was the reason for the failed surgery.

Western Practices

There I was, like any other Western-trained physician, fixated on MRI findings and ignoring other simple explanations that could have caused my symptoms. In my case, the MRI findings took priority over a thorough patient history of illness and a physical examination—two things that any physician should perform. If the physicians who treated me had paid attention to simple details, perhaps my surgery could have been prevented. Just because doctors see everything with definite clarity on an MRI does not mean that they have to ignore other simple causes and jump to conclusions.

Although I was initially against the idea, I saw the best

fix with surgery and went with it. It never crossed my mind that my hand spasm could have been related to something other than my neck compression (cervical spinal stenosis). My colleagues, all doctors with double PhDs and great reputations, convinced me that my neck compression was based on the MRI findings.

In medical school, we were taught that if we listened to a patient's history of his or her illness and completed a physical examination, we could make the diagnosis accurately ninety percent of the time. But unfortunately, this theory has been lost over time because of advances in technology. I was the type of general surgeon who thought that if you had a problem, you could usually fix it or remove it with surgery. It seemed no different than removing the appendix in a case of appendicitis or a colon in the case of colon cancer.

As doctors, we begin to depend on imaging techniques and lab results instead of giving the patient a full evaluation. It makes us lazy. Worst of all, we are taught that most illnesses that cannot be confirmed by our conventional lab tests and elaborate imaging studies do not exist. Still, there are psychosomatic illnesses cannot be confirmed by present-day lab tests and imaging studies. We are simply not that advanced.

Now, if I had viewed medicine in a cognitive way, I would have concluded that my spasms could have been caused by a nerve root or a local muscle problem. I knew, from experience with other physical difficulties, that the cause is often more of a localized problem. For example, when a muscle doesn't get enough circulation, it can go into a spasm or another ailment because it is not getting what it needs.

Too quickly, I jumped at the stenosis diagnosis and went along with the surgery. And when the spasms were still present after the surgery, I was utterly despondent. What a huge risk and expense I had taken for no reason at all! But the ultimate expense was that I had lost what I had loved the most: my career.

It is quite possible that the results of an MRI test will look the same for people who have never had back pain and ones who have chronic back pain. In other words, many people without compression symptoms may still have spinal stenosis.

two

On a Mission

Three years into my retirement and after my surgery, I was invited on a medical mission to Honduras. The week before my trip, I was jogging down a snow-covered road in a park in Colorado. I began to feel extreme fatigue and soreness in my leg muscles that lasted indefinitely.

I got on the plane to Honduras filled with much anxiety, but I was hopeful. I was anxious for several reasons. I was concerned about this new development in my back and legs, and not to mention, I had been away from surgery for three years and I didn't know if I would be as efficient as I once was. I was also anxious about the safety issues in this third world country. Nevertheless, I was excited to be going back into the operating room again, to help people, to be needed again.

The flight was short—just about two hours from Houston. I met a nurse anesthetist from Illinois who had been doing this particular mission for a long time through a Baptist medical group and had a lot of experience with the country. And when we arrived in San Pedro Sula, we rented a car and drove to the mountains. The hospital, built by the Baptist medical group in the 1970s, was located in a remote area of Honduras. After the three-hour drive, we finally made it to the hospital. The drive was terrible on my back and I was quite uncomfortable for most of the ride.

The hospital was one of the most primitive that I had ever seen. It had three operating rooms and most of the patients were placed together in large rooms with several beds. The staff did all of the laundry by hand and hung the clothes outside to dry. The kitchen was also outside and they cooked with firewood.

I was part of a team of about thirty people from all over the United States. Another group came from an Arkansas Baptist church—a physician's assistant and several others who did all the cooking and preparing of the meals for our group. Some even helped in the operating room however they could. There was a fourth-year medical student from the University of Missouri and another general surgeon who came along with his wife. We were lucky to have several nurses with great experience in the operating and recovery rooms.

There were homes next to the hospital for all of us. They had several large rooms with bunk beds, which were very uncomfortable for my back. We had showers but no hot water. It helped that the weather was warm, but it was not warm enough to take cold showers. Unfortunately, the place was also infested with cockroaches.

My first night there was filled with apprehension, which only exacerbated my back condition. I blamed that on the bunk bed. I got up in the middle of the night several times because of the discomfort in my legs. And when I went to the bathroom, I found that several cockroaches had found a home on my toothbrush.

The next morning, when I went to the hospital, I was amazed to see a huge crowd at the doors. People had come from all over Honduras to see the American medical group. Apparently, the news had been broadcast on several television and radio stations and the locals were clearly desperate for good medical care. If we didn't offer it, they'd never received it. We were the only hope they had. Immediately, I forgot all about my back and leg problems. They were no longer my focus. It felt good to be needed, as this was how I had practiced for years.

But I had not done surgery for three years, and I was a bit nervous. I did not know how well I would perform as a surgeon. I hoped surgery would be like riding a bike or swimming because once you learn, you never forget. Then again, I wasn't so sure. The night before, one of the nurses had made a comment about my being away from the operating room that long. In America, if you are away for an extended period of time, they do not let you operate. They call you "out of touch," and you have to go through some training first, like a pilot who has not flown a jet for three years and has to go back to the simulators. In medicine, we do not have simulators or virtual reality surgery—at least not yet.

I walked into the building and up to the front desk in the operating room. I was ready to do whatever they needed. The woman at the desk told me that there were seven gall bladder cases and two thyroid cases. I couldn't believe they had scheduled ten major surgeries for me to do in one day! They told me to do what I could and the rest could be completed the following day.

How could I say no? That word didn't exist for me—it was simply my personality to give as much as I could, even if it meant working long hours without any breaks. A bit reluctant, I started with the first thyroid case of the day. She was a beautiful, nineteen-year-old girl who was extremely apprehensive. A large, firm mass stuck out far on her neck, which felt like cancer to me. There had been no biopsy, x-rays or ultrasound taken on the mass. That technology was simply not available. The only strategy was to take out the mass and send it to a larger center in Honduras for examination. I told her family that it could possibly be cancer and that I would be taking out the entire thyroid gland and some of the lymph glands as well.

The operation began with a long incision in the front of the neck, from side to side. There were three nurses with me during the operation who were all very professional and experienced, which was quite reassuring. It took all of fifteen minutes for me to get back to my previous skill level. It *was* just like riding a bike, and oddly enough, my back pain and the fatigue in my muscles subsided during the surgery.

I removed her entire thyroid gland, which contained the tumor, and closed her up. I went back to her family and gave them the good news. I told them that the entire thyroid gland and some of the lymph glands were removed. And from there on, I felt good. I was starting to feel like my old self again.

I was able to do many surgeries in Honduras. The only thing that helped with my hand spasms was a medication called quinine sulfate. I would not have been able to do any surgeries without this medication. Quinine has many uses, including treating cardiac disease and malaria. It also reduces muscle cramps because it is actually a muscle relaxant.

Despite the numerous lives I impacted and a medical trip that was greatly rewarding, the fatigue and pain continued when I was not in surgery. I started to worry that my symptoms could possibly be those of ALS—amyotrophic lateral sclerosis. The disease is often referred to as "Lou Gehrig's disease." It's the progressive degeneration of the nerve cells, called motor neurons, in the spinal cord and brain, which could eventually lead to paralysis of the muscles. We do not know the exact cause of this disease, but it is eventually fatal.

The other possibility was that I could have had severe nerve root compression due to spinal stenosis. At that time, I knew nothing about tension myositis syndrome or Dr. Sarno's theory on the mind-body interaction. Depriving myself of my own best interests, I developed internal rage. I wasn't even aware of the rage because I had suppressed it for so long. But it all caught up with me. It found a home in my muscles and fascia, and in the nerves in my body. The introverted rage presented itself as chronic pain—what we call myofascial disorder.

If only I had picked up Dr. Sarno's books[1] sooner, I could have prevented a disastrous, life-changing surgery.

three

Spine Surgery

A year and half after my neck surgery, I developed extreme pain in my legs that didn't go away. It felt like I had overworked them when I'd exercised and because of the fatigue in my legs, I experienced difficulty when walking. I immediately thought there was something going on with my back that might be causing the leg problem.

When I came home, I went to the hospital to get another MRI, which showed degenerative disease and spinal stenosis at T10, T12, L2 and L3, combined with the old deformity I had in my lumbar spine.

After reviewing all the x-rays, the spine surgeon determined my symptoms to be caused by the spinal stenosis in my back. The fatigue in my legs was the only symptom I had, other than the pain in my back. I did not have a bowel or bladder problem, which usually necessitate immediate surgery.

Even still, the doctors said there would be a chance that I could get paralyzed from the waist down if I didn't have the surgery. I was shocked beyond belief when they said the word "paralyzed." I had always been such an active person, so paralysis seemed like a death sentence. I didn't understand how this could possibly come about. In repeated physical examinations, I never had any neurological signs or symptoms of myelopathy, an extreme compression of the spinal cord that causes difficulty in walking and coordination.

I consulted three spinal surgeons, only one of which was hesitant about the outcome of such a serious, multiple-fusion surgery. Not one of them mentioned the possibility of a myofascial disorder, which refers to pain and inflammation in the soft tissues or muscles. The possibility of tension myositis syndrome (TMS), named and described by Doctor John Sarno, was never recognized either.

During my illness, medical science didn't understand the cause of tension myositis syndrome (TMS), nor did they know how to cure it. This syndrome has existed since the 1800s, but there was no specific lab test to confirm the disorder. Only a small percentage of doctors recognized the complex clinical conditions of the syndrome. There is no specific lab test to confirm it because our technology is just not that advanced. I had the exact TMS symptoms from A to Z that Dr. Sarno described in his books. It seemed as though I had a classic case of TMS.

The possibility of becoming paralyzed had a huge impact on my life—so much that I needed this problem fixed immediately. I found a spine surgeon with a good reputation in this particular field, and fortunately, there was an opening for the following week.

A few days prior to the spinal fusion surgery, the doctor explained the procedure to me. It entailed opening my abdomen with a twelve-inch incision on my left side, from my belly button to the flank (near the kidneys). During this process, they would have to remove two ribs and part of my pelvic bone and use them for the bone graft. Then, they would open my chest.

The final stage would be to put me on my stomach and open my entire back with a vertical, eighteen-inch incision. In order to fuse eight vertebrae, they would first have to break the deformity at each level of the spine, remove excess bones to make more room for spinal cord and finally put a bone graft and bone cages around and between each vertebra, so they would heal together as a unit. The fusion area was to be held together by rods, plates and screws.

I was extremely wary about their wanting to open my chest. This alone would be a major and risky procedure. From my own experience, I knew that patients who had chest surgery were in considerable pain for a long time. And I had a strong feeling that I would not survive these three procedures at same time. I was now sixty-three years old, and people at that age can only tolerate a certain amount of insult to their system. I told him immediately that I did not want him to open my chest. He agreed, and suggested that perhaps we could get by doing it through the abdomen and back.

The other part that was disturbing was the length of the procedure. He said that if it took more than twelve hours, they would have to close me up and do the rest of the procedure a few days later. I was at a loss either way. I knew that my body would not be able to take the insult of a second surgery and anesthesia a few days later. I had been a surgeon for several years and I knew that some patients my age could tolerate the surgery once, but not a second time. I explicitly said that I would rather have them finish the whole surgery at one time, if that was an option.

The good news was that the surgeon presented my

case at a spine conference and there was a general consensus among the participants that I needed this procedure. I didn't know who these participants were, but I was satisfied to know that other spine surgeons and physicians with similar training agreed with the findings. These doctors all believed in the physical causes of back pain. Each determined most of their diagnoses on MRI findings, and I doubted any of them considered alternative approaches to medical treatment—such a thing was clearly out of the question.

I went through with this horrendous surgery, and I am sorry to say that it did me absolutely no good. In fact, it did a lot of harm.

My Turn on the Firing Line

I woke up on a Tuesday morning at six o'clock. It was May of 2001, and I was in a city far from home. I had found this place through research and was going on the notion that this hospital housed the best spine surgeons in the country.

I got up very early and prepared myself for a rough

day. I took a hot, soapy shower to prevent infection. I had my wife drop me off at the front of the huge teaching hospital with enormous surrounding buildings. It's funny how the grandiose physical appearance of something can give you such a false sense of confidence. I took one look at the fine, big buildings and thought to myself, *How can anything possibly go wrong?*

As a surgeon myself, I knew what complications could arise, but I had confidence that these prestigious doctors and the medical staff would take good care of me. Surely, they would pay extra special attention to a fellow doctor and colleague. Right?

I was scheduled for an 8:00 a.m. surgery. I went in and introduced myself to the staff and filled out the necessary paperwork. I was very anxious. I could still hear the voice of my surgeon ringing in my ear: "If we do not finish in twelve hours, we will close you up and do the rest of the surgery in perhaps four or five days." I was praying that they could just do the whole procedure today.

While I was finishing up my paperwork, I noticed that there were many patients also registering for surgery—several at a time. I felt as though I had just taken a number, like you would at a deli. I was getting more anxious by the minute because I knew the enormity of this surgical procedure. I knew that I could die during or after surgery, or become paralyzed. I asked one of the nurses to give me something to calm my nerves. They placed me on a stretcher and started an IV, and I was better once sedated.

I strongly believe that the patients who are going to have major surgery with a questionable outcome should be given special attention and be separated from the people waiting to have minor procedures. Pre-operative anxiety can have a negative effect on the outcome of the anesthesia and the surgery. These patients, including myself, have different worries and concerns. And, emotionally, they need additional support for the surgery and recovery to go smoothly.

I hadn't been waiting for long when my surgeon came over with the anesthesiologist to see if I had any questions or concerns. The policy of that hospital was that the general surgeon would open the abdomen to create exposure to the spine for the spinal surgeon to begin operating. During this process, the general surgeon would get all of the vital structures, such as major blood vessels, out of the way so the spine surgeon would have easy access to the spine.

I was taken to the operating room, and I can't clearly remember what happened next. My wife told me that the spine surgeon came out of the operating room around ten at night and told her that everything turned out as expected. The operation had taken about twelve and a half hours. He said they'd gotten all eight levels of my spine fused using bone grafts from my pelvis and two ribs that they'd taken out—the most painful part of the procedure. Then, they'd used rods, screws and plates to keep the bone graft in place. The surgeon showed her the x-ray of my spine, which now looked anatomically normal. He told my wife that I would be transferred to the intensive care unit shortly.

I was too unstable to be transferred to the intensive care unit right away. In medical terms, I was what they called "hemodynamically unstable." That means that the patient does not have a stable blood pressure or pulse, could be too heavily dependent on mechanical support or requires a large amount of blood transfusions and fluids. Doctors do not want to transport such patients even short distances because things can go wrong during transport and often, the patients need to be close to the operating room in case they have to go back into surgery.

Into Recovery

Finally, somewhere after midnight, according to my wife, I was transferred from the recovery room to the ICU. This was a small sign of progress because at least I was stable enough to be transferred. However, during the first days in intensive care, I was still unstable. The doctors told my family there was a chance that I may not survive this episode.

I was put on a respirator for the next six days. The reason that doctors place a patient on a respirator is so that the machine can pump air into their lungs. Additionally, during the beginning phases of resuscitation, the patient may have received too much fluid in order to keep their blood pressure up. When there is too much fluid in the lungs, they can become edematous and swollen. In this case, patients are either too weak to breathe on their own or unable to breathe without the machine.

I can remember hearing the nurses telling me to stop trying to talk with the tube in my throat. They even had to restrain my arms because I was constantly trying to bang them against the railings on the sides of the bed. I was so frustrated. It seemed like there was no way I could communicate with them. I needed to tell the nurses I was in a great deal of pain, but I couldn't. It felt like a tractor-trailer had run over my back and crushed all of my vertebrae.

I've always seen myself as someone who has a high threshold for pain. In my twenty-five years of being a surgeon, I had only missed a week of work for an illness. But this, by far, was absolutely the worse pain I'd ever experienced in my life. It wasn't only the pain that bothered me. I could feel a ton of pressure in my abdomen and thighs. The whole thing seemed like some sort of strange sickness that was unfamiliar. Still, to this day, I have a hard time pinpointing an accurate description of the pain.

Later, in the ICU, I developed a pulmonary (lung) infection from a dangerous bacterium. They had to repeatedly suction the secretion from my lungs; otherwise, it would accumulate. The suctioning made me cough violently and aggravated the excruciating pain in my back.

Close to Death

I could clearly hear the doctors and nurses talking about me. They were concerned about my heart because it was beating at a very rapid rate. For someone my age, a rapid heart rate was a warning sign of a possible heart attack. They suspected that the dopamine drip was causing the accelerated heart rate. Dopamine is an IV medication that is used to increase the blood pressure and force the heart to pump more vigorously. In high doses, it can escalate the heart rate at an unsafe pace, but my physicians could not take me off the dopamine because my blood pressure could drop dangerously low.

I can remember how mentally clear I felt that day. I began to think about the patients I'd had during my practice who had attested to becoming "mentally clear" before they'd died. I thought my heart rate was high because I was septic. Sepsis is a condition wherein bacteria toxins fill the bloodstream and cause a series of pathologic, often fatal events. In layman's terms, I thought I had blood poisoning.

After a while, the nurses let my wife come in to visit. She knew I couldn't speak with the tube in my throat so she asked them to give me a piece of paper to write on. I quickly scribbled with my shaky hand, "Transfer me!" I thought the care was inadequate, so I wanted to leave.

"Transfer you? Transfer you where?" she asked.

I didn't answer her, staring off into the distance. She held my hands for a long time. Finally, she said, "I know you are not going to die. I know God has bigger plans for you and you are going to help a lot of people for the rest of your life." My wife looked me straight in the eyes. "I know that for sure and I don't have any doubts."

In that instance, I knew she was right. I could feel this positive energy moving throughout my whole body. I felt the warmth of that energy and miraculously had less pain and fear. A Western-trained doctor could never explain why, suddenly, my heart rate came down and I felt better. In that type of medical training, there simply is no scientific reasoning for it. Western-trained doctors do not subscribe to the mind-body connection of Eastern medicine, so they conveniently called my lowered heart rate a "coincidence."

More Complications

After several long, horrible days, I finally came off the respirator and was able to sustain my own breathing. And shortly after that, I was transferred to the regular floor of the hospital. Against what I had initially thought, the doctors and nurses in the intensive care unit had done a great job of pulling me through the unstable period of my recovery. I'd had exclusive physician care 'round the clock, and without their consistent dedication, I would not be alive today.

Although I was stable, the road ahead was not. The recovery process took me on a whirlwind adventure, and I'm lucky I made it through therapy. I had to wear a brace that started underneath my arms and stopped at my pelvis. I was so weak and debilitated that the slightest exertion—even brushing my teeth—caused severe exhaustion.

Then, one day, I noticed that my abdomen was very

large and bloated. I had not been able to eliminate the gas from my intestines for a few days. As a result of the bloating, my brace became too tight around my abdomen. The doctors ordered an x-ray, and when I saw the results, I knew right away that I had a condition called Ogilvie syndrome, or acute colonic pseudo-obstruction (ACPO), which is a clinical disorder with the signs and symptoms similar to a large bowel obstruction.

This is a condition wherein the large bowel becomes almost paralyzed and loses its movement. Then, the content in the large bowel becomes stagnant and the colon becomes distended, like a balloon, until it finally ruptures. The reasons for this paralysis are often medications, anesthesia or operations on the spinal cord. Sometimes, this also occurs suddenly in the elderly who are in a nursing homes and do not take part in physical activities.

I had seen this condition several times in my own practice. The treatment for Ogilvie syndrome is a drug called neostigmine, which increases the muscle activities of the colon, allowing the material to be eliminated from the bowel. But in my case, because of my recent back surgery, it was not the treatment of choice. I knew I needed to have an immediate colonoscopy to deflate my colon. During a colonoscopy, an instrument with a light at the end of it is inserted into the rectum and advances into the large bowel. This procedure sucks all the air out of the large bowel, deflates the colon, reduces the dilation and stops the possibility of perforation.

I asked to see my general surgeon as soon as possible. He reviewed my x-rays and disagreed with the diagnosis. He said that I just needed some enemas to pass the gas and material from the colon. That entire night, I felt terrible. I was so bloated that I worried my colon would rupture at any moment.

Suddenly, my whole professional life came rushing in front of me like a movie on a big screen. I thought about an eighty-year-old patient from a local nursing home who had come in with the same diagnosis late one night. I'd taken care of his problem right then because I'd known it couldn't possibly wait until the morning. I also remembered several other patients with this problem who I'd taken care of right away unless there'd been a very good reason to wait. My personal plans had never taken priority, nor had the hour of the night become a factor to delay the treatment. This was not the way it should have been. I felt helpless. Cheated, even.

Finally, I asked to talk to my spine surgeon around three o'clock that morning, and explained the situation to him. I told him that I had seen several cases like this during my surgical practice. I told him that in my opinion, I needed a colonoscopy right away because there was a big risk of perforation. I demanded to see a gastroenterologist.

The next morning, a gastroenterologist walked in to my room. The minute I saw this older physician, I knew that he was going to solve my problem. At that moment, I had the same feeling that I'd had when my wife had walked into my ICU room. There was that energy again.

He examined me, looked at the x-ray and agreed with my obvious diagnosis. Twenty minutes later, I was in the operating suite, having my colon deflated with a colonoscopy. When I came out, I felt as if I were a different person. My belly was flat, and I wanted food! And for the first time in forty-eight hours, I ate.

four

Post-operative Care and Rehabilitation

Two weeks after my surgery, I was on my way to a rehabilitation hospital on the opposite end of town. I went into the rehab facility with much hope for my future. It was June, and I was hoping that I would be home and healthy by October, when the trees changed color in Colorado. This season was my favorite time of the year, and I could visualize becoming a normal, pain-free person and enjoying the falling leaves. I could see myself being able to be with my family, jog and get back in shape. All I wanted was my life back.

Before they transferred me to the rehab hospital, they wanted to be sure that I had the insurance to cover the expense. Unfortunately, these days, the economics of medicine can affect patient care. I didn't know what would have happen if I didn't have the financial resources for this service. Luckily, my insurance approved my stay.

The rehabilitation hospital was almost like a very sophisticated nursing home with all the major amenities, including physical and vocational therapy. They even had their own intensive care unit. I was placed in a private room with a window that opened to the parking lot. I could see the outside world and breathe in the fresh air. I was one step closer to my normal life.

Starting Physical Therapy

The physical therapy department was quite excellent. These people were on a mission to undo the havoc that spine surgery had wreaked on my muscles and bones. The physical therapist came into my room, read my chart and gave me a very sympathetic look. She told me she could not believe that a person could go through as much trauma as I had. The eight-level fusion of the spine, using two of my ribs and part of my pelvic bone for the bone graft, seemed like more than any one person could take—not to mention all the hardware holding my spinal column together.

The nurse gave me the initial evaluation and told me what the plan of recovery was, and who my physicians would be. Every morning after breakfast, I was taken to the physical therapy department. This was a huge department with much equipment and apparatuses that were necessary to build back the muscles that the patients had lost. They would also help in increasing the patients' aerobic capacity.

I was assigned to a therapist for evaluation. He designed a specific program to rebuild my muscles and work on the ones that were stiff and inflexible. The aim of therapy was to teach me how to walk again and to show me how to move without putting any stress on the fused area.

Vocational therapy consisted of relearning regular daily activities, from making the bed to cooking. I could not just go and perform these activities as I normally would. I thought I could, but every little thing created extreme fatigue.

The next morning, I was visited by a neurologist who was assigned to care for me. He introduced himself and ran a complete neurological evaluation. The good news was that he did not detect any neurological abnormalities such as nerve or spinal cord damage. I told him that I was experiencing a lot of pain in my back and legs. He increased the dose of narcotic analgesics—my pain medication—and said that if the pain continued, I might benefit from an epidural cortisone injection.

After breakfast, a few attendants got me out of bed and took me to the physical therapy unit. They were amazed when I was able to get out of the bed with very little help. However, after just a few minutes of physical therapy, I felt like I had run a marathon. The effect of the extensive surgery was that my body had to deal with the tremendous feat of healing the bones and surrounding tissue. When I was unable to do anymore of the exercises, they took me back to my room, where I felt as though I drifted into a deep coma for a few hours.

When I awoke that afternoon, a few attendants taught me how to get out of bed alone and go to the bathroom. They showed me new ways of moving that would not put stress on my spine. I had to turn to the right and roll out of bed as one unit, because my back was now like a solid piece of rock. My spine's eight levels were fused together and unable to move separately. Now, I had to treat my back as if it were one whole structure. I could no longer assume that my back had any mobility in the long, fused segment.

A multilevel fusion puts extreme restriction on a patient's life. In experiencing the effects of this surgery, I had to relearn almost every activity and still, there were things that I'd never be able do. Jogging, running, playing tennis and racquetball were completely out of the question. The effects of this operation have been debilitating, in a sense. It is my hope and belief that this operation will one day be considered barbaric and inhumane, and eventually be abandoned.

Waiting to Recover

Lying on my bed, depressed because of my extreme weakness, I was reminded of a question I had asked one of my surgeons before the operation: "How do your patients like this surgery?" He had expressed that patients typically did not like it. I'd assumed that was because patients did not like the post-operative pain and discomfort, and I'd figured it would be a temporary thing. Of course, I realize now that what he was really saying was that patients did not like any part of the outcome of the surgery—not the post-op pain or the healing process.

I was determined to get back to what I'd had before the operation: a normal life. But before I could get too positive, the nurse of another spine surgeon told me that patients are often weak and debilitated for months or years after this kind of surgery. I was officially in for a long, bumpy ride to recovery.

There was a little garden in the rehab unit I was staying in, with flowers and plants. Patients were allowed to go there and sit by the flowers and trees. One day, my wife asked if I wanted to go to the garden, in an attempt to cheer me up. What a great idea! I felt heartened by the fact that this garden existed for patients. It was clear that someone knew the psychology of the people who were recuperating from serious injuries.

I was placed in a reclining chair so that my wife could push me to the garden area. Even that small amount of movement made me exhausted after a few minutes. I had to drink a ton of water and lie down after just a quick visit to the garden.

At this point, I started questioning why this had to happen to me. Because of my medical background, I was well aware of the effects of trauma caused by surgery. But this seemed so different—in fact, far more serious than what I had observed with my own surgical cases. Most of my patients who had had major cancer surgery had recovered in just a few months. Their period of weakness and debilitation had not been as prolonged as mine was becoming.

It is my belief that before the era of modern medicine, surgeons could not have exposed a patient to this much trauma because all of their patients would have died. After we became so medically advanced in intensive care practices, physicians became well-versed in keeping patients alive after major, life-threatening surgeries. What they forgot is how tremendously the patients suffer during and after recovery.

The human body is simply not built to tolerate this much trauma. And the saddest part of all is that a lot of these operations are entirely unnecessary. Medically speaking, the cause of pain is not an anatomical structural abnormality as seen on an MRI. An MRI can be very deceiving. And unfortunately, Western medical practices settle on a diagnosis based on MRI findings, when MRI results are often only the innocent bystanders and not the real causes of the pain.

In the evenings, looking out my rehab room window, I would see patients' families come for visits. I envied all of them because they could walk. They looked so strong and normal. I wished every day that I could be like them. It is amazing how we only appreciate what we have after we've lost it for good. And I'm just as guilty.

The next morning, my therapist decided to take me

out of the building. She said that there were chairs outside to sit on if I got tired. We took the walker and she held me with a belt around my waist, in case I started to fall. We walked toward the doors of the building and went outside.

I asked her, "Do you think that by October, I will be able to walk normally on my own?" October was four months away.

She was silent for a moment, and then she smiled. "I don't see any reason why not," she said. It was the first glimpse of hope.

Insurance Dictates Discharge

I had officially been in the rehab for three weeks. I'd lost a tremendous amount of weight, and my brace had to be adjusted on weekly basis. By this time, I could walk and get in and out of the bed without too many difficulties. But I quickly learned that when a patient can walk again, insurance companies kick the patient right out of the rehab unit. They dictate to the doctors what patients need to be discharged, and take no responsibility for the outcome of their recovery. It was decided that I would be transferred from the rehab unit to a motel room—authority without responsibility.

My wife picked me up from the rehab and drove to the motel. Sitting upright in the car on the way to the motel was very difficult. I felt every bump in the road during the twenty-minute ride, and when we arrived, it was a relief. That evening, my wife took me next door, to a restaurant, for dinner. I was unable to sit up for very long and had to return to my room shortly after our meal. Every night, I was miserable with pain and I kept sedating myself with medication just to get by.

I had one more appointment with my spine surgeon before I could go home. At his office, the technicians took x-rays. The spine surgeon reviewed them with me and he was quite proud of how good my spine looked. It was clear that I did not have any more deformity in my spine and that the normal curvature was present. I felt like I was a mess, but at least my spine looked great.

I had a lot of pain in my back that had not been there before the surgery. I also had a new pain in my legs, and my toes were numb. I was so weak and debilitated that I felt helpless. I asked the surgeon when he thought I would feel normal again, and he mentioned that I would probably be able to drive in about four more weeks.

five

Going Home

The next day, my wife and I flew home. There was no way I would be able to sit comfortably in a coach seat, so I had to take first class to be able to recline. The trip home was a huge physical undertaking for both my wife and me, but I was fortunate to be going home and getting well again. Unfortunately, my body had plans other than healing during the next several months.

My wife and I got off the airplane at Denver International Airport, and a wheelchair was waiting for me. I felt a little ashamed to sit in a wheelchair. I was self-conscious, and felt as if everyone in the airport was looking at me. It was hard to get in the wheelchair because I was wearing the brace, which covered most of my upper torso.

Finally, we got to the baggage claim, where my daughter was waiting for us, and fortunately, it did not take too long to get our bags and to get the car. As soon as I sat down in the passenger seat, I felt exhaustion overcome me. It had been brewing those long three hours on the airplane.

When I arrived home, there was a hospital bed for me in the living room, next to the television. It felt so good to be home. And I think my dogs were just as happy to see me as I was to see them! The first night sleeping in my own home was great, but the pain after the long trip was tremendous. I was only able to sleep periodically and had to wake up every hour to take more medication.

I should have been informed that life is very different after a major spinal fusion, especially for someone who is over sixty years old. The fact is that spinal fusion, in most cases, will not relieve the pain—one major fact left out when I was signing the surgery consent form. It is a tremendous effort to get back to a relatively normal life after such a major operation. It took me five years of tremendous efforts to get back to my normal life, and I am proud of it. However, there are many who cannot get past their post-operation tribulations and even end up in wheelchairs.

Major spinal fusion may alleviate and correct some

of your problems, but it will ultimately create ten other abnormalities in your kinetic and daily functioning. I am sure that there are many statistics that can repudiate what I am saying, but we are patients, not statistics. There are so many who share my story.

My good friend, a radiologist, had a spinal fusion on his neck and ended up with such severe, chronic pain that he had to retire from his profession. I took care of him after the surgery and I thought his pain was an unfortunate exception to the success of the surgery. The operation changed his life and ended his profession at a very young age. I can remember him telling me how he had never been told about the possibility that this could happen to him.

An Uncertain Future

It was June in Colorado—one of the best times of year to be there. But all I could look at was my body in the bathroom mirror. I was shocked at how much weight I had lost. I was all skin and bone, and I could practically count every rib in my torso. I was devastated by my appearance and had no relief from the horrible pain. No one deserved this kind of surgery. It was so inhumane. I began to feel this incredible anger toward the people who had exposed me to this kind of misery.

The pain continued on daily basis. From the time I woke up until I went to bed, I was in pain. Strangely enough, the tenderness in my back and legs was not the kind of hurting I'd experienced before the surgery. It was completely new. I could see that I had traded my relatively fair condition before surgery for a new, debilitating condition. I knew I had made a huge mistake.

Only one of the spine surgeons had officially told me that I could become paralyzed. And when I'd asked my treating surgeon about paralysis, he had not ruled out the possibility, but had stayed quiet about it. I'd always felt that there was a chance, but if I hadn't gotten better with physical therapy and spinal injections, surgery would have to be the next step.

I felt very insecure about my future and about the quality of my life going forward. I discovered that this insecurity develops with chronic pain. We do not know where the origin of pain is or where it is coming from, and we do not know how long it is going to last. My fear was that I was going to feel this way until the end of my life. I was terribly nervous that I may be dependent on pain medication for the rest of my life and was uncertain about my future.

Playing the Pain Medication Game

I was going through all of my pain medication rather quickly. And when I called my surgeon's office about receiving more medication, they told me I would have to find a pain clinic locally to have the medications renewed. Luckily, they were kind enough to give me a limited supply until I could get an appointment with another physician.

But unfortunately, getting an appointment with a pain clinic is easier said than done. Often, you have to wait a minimum of a month to be seen. Pain clinics are in such demand because there is an epidemic of chronic pain in this country. It is my belief that the incidence of chronic pain after spine surgery is unbelievably high. More specifically, the pain clinics are overwhelmed with spinal surgery patients, and most of them didn't even need the surgery in the first place. And when the surgery didn't help them, they were referred to a pain clinic

A high percentage of all back surgeries fail to solve the original problem—quite an alarming figure, wouldn't you say? Thousands of people are added to the failed back surgery list every year and most of them become disabled for the rest of their lives. These people are usually referred to other specialists when their pain continues and spend an additional small fortune to get better.

Going through bottles of pain killers every few weeks, I didn't know how I would manage without them. My wife suggested I see our local doctor. I knew the woman was a caring physician, so we called and I got an appointment for the next day.

six

Surgery...All for Nothing?

The nurse called my name and I entered the back office. She checked my vital signs and weight—a minuscule 120 pounds—and said I looked debilitated, but assured me that this was common for people who'd had a spinal fusion. It was a bit comforting to know that I wasn't an exception.

I sat on the exam table until the doctor came in. Maria was a kind woman who took the time to examine me and look at my x-rays. And for the first time since I'd become ill, I saw a sympathetic face. She actually listened. Instead of just looking at my MRI, she gave me a complete physical exam and looked over my medical history. I was finally a patient again, and not just the Social Security number on my chart.

Maria was what a professional physician should be. She refilled my pain medications and gave me the confidence that she cared about my condition. And at the end of my visit, she reassured me that I would not feel like this forever. I left her office knowing that I had adequate medical support. No longer did I have to suffer.

It is my belief that medical professionals have forgotten how to "touch" their patients. It is true that physicians do not have enough time to communicate with every patient on a personal level. But the power of touch in the healing process is essential. After my visit with my local physician, I felt as though I had a fighting chance. I also found an anesthesiologist who specialized in pain management and made an appointment to see him in a month. Perhaps he could use his expertise to lower my pain level.

Chronic pain is an illness that is often misunderstood. When pain lasts for a long time, it has a tendency to destroy the life of a person. It erodes the confidence of even the strongest human beings. My whole life and each day's events became centered around how much pain I was in. And I knew this was no way to live.

Because my appointment with the pain management specialist was a month away, I saw my family doctor in the meantime. At my visit, she told me that I might have to be on narcotic medications for the rest of my life. She mentioned that she treated many people in my situation and usually, lifelong meds were the outcome. I couldn't accept spending the rest of my life sedated—this was not an option.

Nothing Is Working!

It was a long month, waiting for my appointment with the pain specialist. Finally, the day arrived. I entered the pain center with much anticipation. And as I walked to the registration desk with much hope for my medical future, there was no warmth from the receptionist. The staff at the desk did not pay any attention to the people who came in, nor did they even glace up at me when I arrived.

The pain center was in a hospital building as an outpatient clinic. I tried to shrug off the cold receptionist and sat in the waiting room with my hope intact. This doctor was specialized in pain—surely, he could help. Even if he could *reduce* my pain, it would be worth it.

A nurse came into the waiting room and escorted me to a typical, cold examination room. I immediately liked the nurse. She was a middle-aged, compassionate woman. It seemed as if she didn't fit in with this cold institution.

During my examination, she paid attention to every detail. She noticed that my breathing was not very deep. My breath didn't come from my diaphragm. I could see it in her face that she herself had been through the same pain and suffering in her lifetime. I believed that she had felt what I had been going through for the last several months.

Shortly after that, Dr. Jay arrived. He was a middle-aged anesthesiologist, sophisticated and moderately professional. However, he did not treat me like a colleague. He completely ignored the fact that I was a doctor. But I didn't let it bother me; I just prayed that he would find the source of my pain and do something about it.

After a brief exam, he suggested that I might benefit from a series of epidural injections. What this meant was that I would be receiving a spinal injection of corticosteriods and Novocain into the space around the spinal cord, or the epidural space. The hope was that the injections would reach the nerve roots, which might have been inflamed or compressed by scar tissue.

Dr. Jay did not come up with any definite diagnosis of

my condition, but he was willing to help. I consented to the procedure even though there was only a twenty-percent chance that the epidural injections would help me. It was better than no chance at all.

Dr. Jay decided that it was best to have the first injection during that initial visit. Because he preferred to perform the procedure under sedation, an IV was inserted into my arm.

A new nurse came in to give me the IV. Apparently, the other nurse had been pulled out of the office during my visit to go to another department. To me, this was a complete interruption of patient care. The new nurse did not know anything about me. She was there to start the IV and nothing else. She prepared the IV and had trouble sticking the needle in my veins several times. I knew why she kept missing the vein and I made a comment as to how she could better use the needle. She didn't appreciate my advice. Finally, they called some else in to start the IV.

Eventually, I had my epidural injection and left the hospital building. My chronic pain was temporarily gone. It was invigorating not to have pain for the first time, and I was almost in a state of euphoria. But, unfortunately, the pain came back after just a few hours, once the effect of the local anesthetic wore off. I did not lose faith, however. I knew that sometimes, it could take more than three injections for the pain to dissipate.

Every two weeks I saw Dr. Jay and had repeated epidural injections with no lasting success. And, sometimes, when I left his office, I felt that the treatments even made the pain much worse.

Seeing no clear results, Dr. Jay suggested increasing my pain medications, which included heavy doses of oxycodone. I took his suggestion and took more pain medication every day. Unfortunately, I developed sleep apnea, which is one of the side effects of oxycodone. This forced me to sleep with equipment called a CPAP (continuous positive airway pressure), so that I could breathe properly in my sleep. Essentially, Dr. Jay did nothing for me except over-drug me with pain medication.

A few weeks later, I called one of my colleagues. She had a huge practice in Southern California and I knew she specialized in physical therapy and rehab medicine. I wanted to get her opinion. In our phone conversation, she suggested that I see a pain specialist in Colorado who happened to be one of her students. She spoke very highly of this physician and thought she could help me.

I took her recommendation and the next thing I knew, I was sitting in yet another pain clinic, waiting to see a physician who was a physiatrist—a physical therapy specialist. My colleague had raved about her. She had been trained in one the best centers in the country and had a terrific reputation for knowing the new techniques in pain management.

She immediately ordered a complete x-ray evaluation of my spine, including a myelogram, in which they inject die into the spinal canal to see the details in the nerve roots and spinal cord. My results came back normal. I found I was not suffering from any compression on the spinal cord or on any specific nerve root. It was apparent that the spine surgeon had done a good job in curing the spinal stenosis that had been there prior to surgery.

Based on the distribution of pain in my legs, the doctor suggested a series of nerve root injections with cortisone. I wasn't ready for this. I was skeptical of having another round of injections, and I needed time to think.

It was November—four months after my surgery. The x-ray of my spine showed that the bone graft was working and the fusion was becoming solid. My surgeon gave me permission to take the brace off, but I continued with the physical therapy. And, unfortunately, the physical therapy made my body feel much worse.

There was too much evidence that my back pain was not caused by structural abnormality, and I was beginning to realize that my surgery may have been completely unnecessary. After I began to research the unconventional causes of back pain, I became more convinced that my chronic pain was probably originating from the muscles and fascia, and not from the structural abnormalities of the spine. Could I have really gone through all that surgery for nothing?

seven

Alternative Therapies

I started to lose my faith in traditional medicine. I decided to try alternative therapies because I was becoming so desperate. In my own research, I came across an acupuncturist. She came to my home and performed several sessions of acupuncture, but unfortunately, her therapy didn't do anything for me.

I also signed up for a seminar on alternative and holistic methods specifically for physicians. During these meetings, I met several physicians who had different approaches toward treating chronic illnesses. It was there that my outlook changed on medicine. I was shocked to learn just how inadequate Western medicine was in treating chronic illness. And during my thirty years of practice, it had never once crossed my mind that American physicians were not experienced in this type of treatment.

As a Western physician, I had a mentality like most doctors—that we could treat chronic illnesses as if they were acute illnesses. But now, I was a prime example of the failure of Western medicine, and there were millions of people suffering from the same misdiagnoses and improper treatment. I believe that this is one of the reasons why we are becoming a nation of disabled people.

I became obsessed with educating myself on these alternative medical approaches. I took courses and seminars on the science of energy medicine, mind-body medicine, homeopathic medicine, traditional Chinese medicine, Ayurvedic medicine, spiritual healing, manual medicine and the therapeutic effects of yoga and Chi Chong. The alternative medicine course was taught by one of the most brilliant physicians I had ever met in my career, and the environments at these conferences were refreshing. I felt as though I belonged to a group—one that cared for the wellbeing of the sick.

I learned that pain was a lesson instead of purely an enemy. And years later, after the seminars, I noticed that my own pain and suffering were my biggest lessons in medicine.

Holistic medicine treats the entire person—the mind, body and spirit. One of the main goals of holistic medicine is for the patient to be completely content and blissful. Essentially, contentment is ignored in Western medicine, and instead, lack of illness is considered "good health." If someone has a heart attack today, it in no way represents that he was healthy yesterday. Western medicine will tell you differently.

In relation to my own pain, the negative thoughts I was having definitely increased the level of my pain significantly. Sometimes, I wondered if the cause of my pain was really structural abnormalities, or just negative emotions making the pain worse.

In the conferences that I attended, Dr. Robert Keck, MDiv, PhD, noted that a spiritual relationship with God or a higher power is an additional factor in healing chronic illness and pain. And in recent years, our society has been paying more attention. I also learned that a spiritual relationship with God or a higher power is an additional reason for and factor in healing chronic pain and illness. I believe that this strong relationship creates a mystifying power that can bring a long-lasting "blissful environment," as Dr. Candace Pert called it. This new, heavenly environment changes the body's chemistry, and illnesses and pain have a hard time living in that sort of body milieu.

It is now time for us to reach new, miraculous heights in the healing arts. Like poet David Whyte said, we must "find ourselves opening to the life we have refused again and again until now." Emmet Fox, the outstanding spiritual teacher, once said, "Whatever you believe with feeling, *that* is what you bring into your life."

In my experience with my own patients, I had taken care of a large number of people who had been critically ill with multifaceted and complex medical problems. I had noticed that patients who had strong relationships with God, or even strong bonds with their communities and families, had had successful recoveries.

According to many scientific studies, people who have less contact with friends and relatives, church memberships, groups and organizations had three times the overall death rate than those who are connected with other people. And women with breast cancer have twice the death rate if they have no support system. There have also been studies that suggest that massage therapy increases the immune function of AIDS patients. Individuals with AIDS, cancer, back pain and other severe medical conditions that are hard to cure with conventional medical therapies often seek out these types of alternative therapies.

Because of my several failed attempts to rid my body of pain, I knew that I was one of those patients who could not be helped by conventional medicine. Just ten years before, if someone had asked me about alternative and holistic medicine, I would have laughed at the concept. Now, I was desperate.

In my research, I came across energy medicine healers. These healers are highly spiritual people who work on a totally different paradigm. I met with three energy healers and received a treatment called "healing touch" from two of them.

Lisa, a healer and a registered nurse, started a series of treatments with me at her office. I would lie on my stomach on the examining table and feel heat coming from her hands. It was incredible. Sometimes her hands were as far as six inches from the surface of my back. My pain was lessened immediately, and I felt an enormous sense of relief. It was if a 200-pound weight had been lifted from my body. Originally, I'd thought she had placed a heating pad on my back, but she had not used any tools whatsoever—just her hands.

The energy coming from her soothed my back. I wanted the sessions to last forever. It was a nurturing energy therapy. "Healing touch" influences and adjusts the body's energy field and supports a patient's natural ability to heal. Its practitioners are able to see the energy—

an aura—around people and other living things. Sometimes, they can see that the flow of energy is obstructed or disturbed. When Lisa ran her hands around my back, she detected where the flow of energy was disturbed. It stopped at the source of my pain.

I felt great after the treatments, but my relief never lasted longer than a twenty-four-hour period. The pain always came back, but for the whole day, my endorphin level was high, and I was in a good mood. The energy treatments gave me hope for the future and I knew that I was on my way to living pain-free.

I was deprived of life's effortless enjoyments, and it killed me. Sleeping, enjoying a good meal in a restaurant, going to movie, reading a book or taking a walk were all struggles for me. Knowing that I had trouble with simple activities turned me into a pessimistic person. With much free time on my hands, I began to search the Internet. In chat rooms and on pain Web forums, I found many people in similar situations as myself. In some ways, it was comforting to know that I was not the only unfortunate one.

My fellow colleagues and the doctors I respected the most had failed me completely. My health was declining, and I had more problems than when I had originally sought help. Each physician I trusted with my life had simply walked away from my worsening situation. They had all made me feel as though my chronic pain was my own fault, and as though their methods of treatment had nothing to do with it. I had never imagined that I would have to seek treatment on my own, especially after spending countless hours in surgery and in recovery. But if I was going to get my life back, it was my only choice.

eight

Back to the Surgeon

In December of 2001, about six months after my surgery, I went back to my surgeon, to tell him about my miserable condition. Although I hadn't had much success with conventional medicine, part of me still believed he could help me.

Before my visit, I had informed them about my chronic pain so they knew that I'd had several unfavorable results. I arrived at the office hoping that my surgeon could find a way to diagnose the cause of my pain. The environment was cold and unwelcoming. The nurse was quiet, and she didn't seem like the same person she had been prior to surgery. It made me feel guilty that I'd ended up with a bad outcome, but maybe it was a reaction. Perhaps they were feeling guilty too.

The surgeon thoroughly examined me and looked at my x-ray charts. He explained that the pain could either be coming from the facet back joints of the spine or from a herniated disc. He suggested that I see a pain specialist who was very good at dealing with patients with similar problems. The office called and arranged an appointment for me.

I left the office a bit aggravated and went to the pain clinic the next day. The pain specialist suggested a series of corticosteroids injections around the nerve roots. He recommended a group of physicians who would be able to see me in Denver. I immediately called the office when I got home and set up an appointment a month later.

By the end of January, I was sitting in the office of the pain specialist. He specialized in spinal injections and I was hoping he could help me get rid of my chronic pain. I was starting to run out of options. I waited for him in the exam room, and a young physician walked in. He listened to my history, took my packet of x-rays, asked me about the location of my pain and scheduled my nerve root injection sessions. Not once did he examine me or even look at my x-rays.

As I waited for the nurse to schedule an appointment for me, I watched the young doctor dictate my record for more than ten minutes. I realized that the quality of the patient medical records were more important than the quality of patient care. After all, insurance companies and the government demand a perfect medical record.

I am not criticizing this young physician—the error is in the system. Suddenly, I remembered back to when I'd started my practice in a 200-bed hospital. There had only been a staff of four who had taken care of the medical records. These girls had been occasionally busy, but had plenty of time to do their work. When I had retired twenty-five years later, the hospital had been reduced to 100 beds, and the medical record department had a staff of ten who were always behind with the documents. As a physician, I felt that medical records stole valuable time from patients and reduced the quality of care.

The day came for my injections, and I signed in with the ambulatory surgery center. I had my first nerve root injection and went home hopeful that it would work. Unfortunately, the pain got worse for a few days, but I still hoped that after the treatment, my medical benefits would kick in. But that, of course, never happened.

When I spoke to the doctor about my additional pain, he increased my narcotic medication and made another suggestion. He recommended a radiofrequency ablation of my sensory nerves down to the facets, which are the back part of the spine articulation. In this procedure, called a rhizotomy, the spines articulate with each other in the back. If these joints become involved with arthritis and their surfaces become rough and irregular, the spinal movement can cause pain. The radio frequency kills the sensory nerves that are attached to these facets so that the patient does not feel pain. Radio frequency waves are like radio waves. They generate heat and destroy the nerve.

I can only imagine what that treatment would cost my insurance company. Certainly, it wouldn't be cheap. But at that point, I didn't care about the cost. I was ready to pay anything to feel better.

Minimally Invasive Surgery

In the spring and summer of 2002, I was completely fed up with conventional treatment for pain. I was put on heavy doses of Neurontin and narcotic analgesics, which made me extremely tired. They might as well have just given me a death sentence.

Through my Internet research, I read about minimally

invasive surgery of the spine. This is a technique wherein surgery is done by inserting a tiny video camera through puncture holes instead of a large incision, allowing the surgeon to look at the operative field on a television screen. This procedure is similar to removing someone's gall bladder with a laparoscope. The difference between regular surgery and minimally invasive surgery, regarding post-operative pain, is tremendous. Usually, the patient can go home right after surgery instead of having to stay in the hospital for several days at a time.

I saw this as a much kinder, more humane option. As a general surgeon, I had performed this kind of surgery on hundreds of patients. In my experience, the outcome had almost always been very rewarding for them. But the drawback to this kind of surgery is the learning curve. The amount of study and practice to master this type of technique can take a long time. The problem is that the camera offers the surgeon no depth perception. The images are only two-dimensional, so it is hard to get used to it.

Sadly, this kind of surgery is not offered to spine surgeons during their training. For this reason, many of them do not believe in minimally invasive surgery. In 1989, when a gall bladder was first removed by laparoscopy, it was heavily criticized by all the big names in surgery. But following the first operation, laparoscopic surgery spread like wildfire. Patients started demanding it in opposition to making a seven-inch incision in the abdomen. In just eighteen months, laparoscopic surgery became the standard procedure for gall bladder removal. Perhaps, one day, spine surgery will go through the same changes and minimally invasive surgery will be the norm.

I found a few places in this country that performed minimally invasive spine surgery. There were many places in Europe and South America that offered the procedure, but the two centers I called in the United States had experience with thousands of cases. The institute I chose had resources for patients who came from all over the world. They helped patients find the right hotels or an apartment to stay in before and after the surgery.

Prior to my visit in June 2002, I was seen by neurologists and internal medicine practitioners, and had many x-rays and MRIs in the same institute. By the time I was set to have my surgery, everything was ready for the head surgeon to review.

nine

Learning to Deal With Chronic Pain

After six minimally invasive surgeries, I still had pain in my back. The surgeries released all the scar tissue in my back, burned and destroyed all sensory nerves that were connected to the facet joints and even took out some of the screws and plates that were pressing on the nerves. The pain level did go down, but it was still present. Eventually, it came back with the same intensity. I wondered if it was the placebo effect—if a patient believes that the procedure is going to help the pain, it will happen. But, usually, it does not last. In some cases, the placebo effect even stops the progress of cancer in some patients on temporary basis.

But I just had to face it: Pain was my constant companion. Patients in chronic pain often become depressed, isolated, lonesome and, at times, very angry. I was going through all these stages. And on the top of that, I was beginning to lose mobility.

Meanwhile, I noticed a protrusion in the left side of my abdomen and flank that was gradually getting worse. I knew it was not a hernia or rupture of the muscles or fascia in this part of my abdomen. It was because of a nerve injury to a muscle called the transversus abdominis—an inner, muscular layer of the abdomen that holds all the internal organs together like a belt. If the nerve to this muscle is cut, then the muscle becomes paralyzed and cannot hold the internal organs. Instead, they bulge out.

I wondered if this was the cause of my chronic pain. If the transversus is not functioning properly, it makes the other internal muscles around the spine work harder. As a result, these muscles are overworked and go into spasms that can cause severe pain.

I tried to research the effect of paralysis on the transversus, but I could not find any literature on it. There was a lot of information about the significance of the transversus in the stabilization of the back, but nothing specifically regarding the paralysis of one side of this muscle, or if it could be the cause of significant back pain.

I consulted a general surgeon who often opened the

abdomen for spine surgeons who were performing spinal fusions. He said that he had seen many patients who'd had the spinal fusion surgery walking around with bulges in their bellies, but he did not think that it could be the cause of my back pain.

During this time, I had been seeing a physical therapist twice a week and doing exercises at home on regular basis. The only thing that helped me, if only for a few hours, was the trigger-point release on my gluteus muscles. The therapist would apply pressure on the muscles, which were rigid and knot-like, until they released and became relaxed. I loved it because it released the pressure and the knots in the gluteus muscles, which allowed me to move around much easier. However, despite the relief, the exercises made me extremely sore. I decided to discontinue physical therapy and do mild exercises and daily walking on my own.

The Pump

On the recommendation of my primary doctor, I decided to go to a different pain management physician. I heard about something called the "pain pump," which was developed by the Medtronic Company. Many said it was a very effective pain reliever for the back. The pump is implanted under the skin over the abdomen. They put a small tube around the spinal cord in the back and connect the tube to the pump. The pump automatically infuses small amounts of medication (like morphine) around the spinal cord. So, instead of taking large amounts of medication by mouth, the pump delivers minute amounts of medication to the local area of the spinal cord pain and the nerve roots.

Unfortunately, there is a possible, dangerous side effect with this system: The tube around the spinal cord could cause scar tissue if left in place for an extended period of time.

My thinking was, if I could have this device implanted for six months and be on my way to being pain-free, I would have ample time to be active and build up my core muscles to better support my back. Then, I would have the pump removed. The thought of having less pain, even for six months, gave me high expectations.

My new pain management doctor knew how to implant these pumps and had performed many such operations on other patients. After a few days, I was able to make an appointment with him. I went in, filled out the forms, and waited for my name to be called.

The physician was very understanding. He examined me and thought I would be a great candidate for the pump. He discussed the lists of medications that could be administered through the pump, and some of them had proven to be quite effective. But prior to the pump implantation, I needed to be evaluated by a psychologist. The doctor gave me the name of a psychologist, but they warned me that they did not accept my insurance or Medicare, so I would have to pay for it out of my pocket. I didn't care how much it cost. I was ready to pay anything for something promising.

I took a two-hour test before seeing the psychologist. After examining me, he concluded that I did not have any psychological problems. The psychologist gave me the name of an acupuncturist who could help me in the meantime. Even though I had tried acupuncture before and found it not helpful, I was willing to see this new Chinese acupuncturist. Soon after, I began five sessions of treatment with no noticeable effects.

After a few weeks, I saw my pain specialist and hoped he would schedule me for the pump implantation. He said that the next step was to get the help of a spine surgeon to put the catheter and tube around my spinal cord. I still had a lot of hardware in my back, which the spine surgeon would have to remove to create room for the insertion of the catheter. Quite reluctantly, I made an appointment with the spine surgeon that he recommended and went to his office with all of my x-rays in hand.

He looked at my x-rays and then took some new ones. After he looked at the x-rays, he told me that I'd developed spodylolisthesis in the remaining portion of my lumbar spine, and I needed to fuse the rest of my back. I couldn't believe it! He did no physical examination; there was no history to my pattern of pain or its location. The decision was made purely on x-ray findings. I was appalled that he would subject me to yet another enormous operation so quickly. I was a physician and I knew my anatomy. I knew that the locations of the pain in my legs and groin were inconsistent and did not match my x-ray findings. Anatomically, it was a totally incorrect diagnosis because the pain was in the wrong location. When I came out of that office, my pain level had skyrocketed to the highest levels.

I remembered all too well the people I'd met at the minimally invasive spine surgery center who'd had multiple open surgeries, continued to get worse and ended up in a wheelchair.

When I went back to my pain specialist, I was very angry. He completely catered to the opinion of the spine surgeon and accepted his opinion blindly. After I told him what had happened, he suggested that I see another spine surgeon for a second opinion.

So I did. The second spine surgeon did not recommend another surgery, but he was not very accepting of the idea of a pain infusion pump. I had a hard time finding a spine surgeon to remove the hardware so I could get the infusion pump, and so I never got it. I was back to square one—again.

ten

Not Giving Up

One day, it came to me. What about the Mayo Clinic, the Cleveland Clinic or The Spine Center at Johns Hopkins? I found their Websites and discovered that they had nothing new to offer but the same old, traditional medicine options I had been stuck with for so long. At that point, I really gave up. I knew that what they would do would be a repetition of my past experiences.

In searching for treatments other than conventional medicine, I heard about treating chronic back pain with prolotherapy. It sounded scientific and it made sense. The first part of the word, "prolo," comes from "proliferation," which is the growth of cells and tissues. Medications, which are irritants, are injected into weak ligaments or connective tissues that have been damaged. It makes them grow stronger so they can support the spine.

Ligaments are connective tissue structures much like rubber bands, which hold two adjacent bones. If they become damaged, they cannot hold the bones together, in turn causing abnormal, painful motion. Injection of the irritant into this tissue gives the body the message that it was injured. The body then starts putting out healing material, such as collagen, to strengthen the ligament. It takes at least a month for this process to take place.

This treatment is used for sport injuries, chronic back pain, arthritis and fibromyalgia. The irritant, which is injected into these tissues, is like sugar water or phenol and a variety of other solutions. It causes a strong, local, inflammatory reaction, which stimulates the body's own healing reaction.

I found a physician who practiced prolotherapy on daily basis. He'd had a good rate of success with this treatment, and had patients flying in from all over to seek his advice. My impression from the first interview was that he had a good knowledge of anatomy, especially that of the spine, muscles and fascia around it. The doctor was also involved in teaching this discipline to other physicians all over the country.

After my initial evaluation, he thought I would benefit from injections in the lower spines. The x-rays showed that my lower spines were not as stable and that one vertebra had slipped slightly in front of the other. It was the same diagnose the surgeon for the pump had given me: spodylolisthesis. In my case, there was a forward displacement of L4 over the L5.

The physician also thought that the joint between sacrum, the end of the spine, and the ilium, the bones of the pelvis, was unstable. Strong ligaments hold the sacrum and the ilium together. If the ligament becomes too thin or weak, the joint has too much movement, causing excessive pain.

On his recommendation, I went through several sessions of prolotherapy injections, which was extremely painful. These treatments are not for the weak. It takes a lot of stamina to tolerate the pain. When the doctor pushed with his thumbs on the weak areas, I could feel an exaggerated form of the exact pain I'd had all day. Despite this treatment, several months of therapy did not help me.

It was time for me to accept my state in life—one of chronic pain and disability. The problem was that I just couldn't. There had to be a solution.

eleven

Finding My Own Solution

Years later, after my second surgery, I realized that when I drank a lot of water, my spasms went away. It was so simple! For two months, I drank water very regularly, at least eight glasses a day, and it made the spasms completely go away.

Then, I came across an excellent book called *Your Body's Many Cries for Water* by Dr. F. Batmanghelidj. It talked about hydration and how the body cries out for water in many different ways. Dr. Batmanghelidj wrote that because over time, humans gradually lose their thirst sensation, our bodies become chronically and increasingly dehydrated from an early adult age. We develop a water deficiency just as we do any other vitamin or mineral deficiencies as we age.

My research brought me to conclude that it was chronic dehydration of my hand muscles that made the spasms happen in the first place. Those were the muscles I used the most. If I had been a runner, I would have been getting spasms in my legs. Every day, I drink water; otherwise, the spasms will come back.

I also came to believe that the chronic dehydration growing worse each year was a major factor in my back pain. Years of dehydration had caused the same kind of spasms to occur in my back and leg muscles. When I was a physician, some of the older patients complained of spasms in their hands and leg muscles, and I gave them medications to reverse the condition. At the time, it didn't cross my mind that these patients were chronically dehydrated.

It is important to read all you can about back pain before you consent to any procedure. Dr. John Sarno's four books—*The Mindbody Prescription, Healing Back Pain, Mind Over Back Pain* and *The Divided Mind: The Epidemic of Mindbody Disorders*—changed my life, and I believe that everyone with chronic back pain should read them.

Dr. Sarno is a professor of clinical rehabilitation medicine at New York University. He created a revolutionary program that has helped thousand of patients overcome their back problems. During many years of practice, taking care of people with chronic back and neck pain, he discovered that the causes of most back pain are tension and suppressed emotions. It is from a condition he calls tension myositis syndrome (TMS).

Tension, which is repressed emotion and anger, can cause decreased blood flow to muscles and fascia (a band of dense, soft tissue that surrounds and envelopes the muscles) or spinal nerves, creating a painful condition. TMS can target any muscle or nerve in the body and create symptoms that mimic diseases that are caused by structural abnormalities. It can affect any age group, including children.

These books changed my thinking process regarding the cause of pain. They created a paradigm change, which turned things around and gave me some hope. The strange thing is that I don't even remember how I came across these books. Perhaps it was while researching chronic pain on the Internet. I remember being tired and frustrated with my research on my usual medical sites and in conventional text books. Nothing came up that was useful to me until I found these books.

Dr. Sarno has successfully treated over 30,000 people

with chronic back and neck pain. He has concluded that the cause of most chronic pain is not the structural abnormalities that we see on CAT scans and MRIs; instead, it is psychosomatic in nature, due to repressed emotions—rage, anger and depression—in the subconscious mind.

Psychosomatic illnesses are not mental disorders; rather, they are normal occurrences between the mind and body. And mind-body interaction is not a mental disorder; it is completely normal. If we repress anger or any other unpleasant emotions, the emotion will get buried in the subconscious mind. We are not aware of the suppressed rage in the subconscious mind until the emotion tries to escape into the conscious mind, appearing in the form of physical symptoms. We in turn feel the physical repercussions (i.e,. back pain, neck pain, leg and arm pain and spasms.)

The mind believes that the back or neck pain is less of a threat than the emotional rage that is trying to surface to the conscious mind. Thus, the mind develops physical symptoms in the body as a protective mechanism, to prevent suppressed emotions from entering into the conscious state. The mind cuts down the circulation to the nerves and muscles, creating severe pain. Usually, these symptoms occur where there was once an old injury or structural problem to make a potential condition believable.

Dr. Sarno did not use any medications or procedures to cure his patients. He just gave them knowledge. And the knowledge was the permanent cure. However, if patients did not respond to his treatment or their symptoms were extremely severe, he would send them for psychotherapy.

Although he has helped several thousand people, Dr. Sarno's theory about TMS is often not recognized by Western medicine because it cannot be proven in a lab. Because his study is based on the interaction of the mind and body, there are no test-tube experiments or imaging techniques to solidify his concept. And unfortunately, because they are uninformed, doctors often dismiss TMS as a possible cause of chronic pain. It is amazing what the mind can do. It can cause huge changes in the chemistry of the body, and the body has an overwhelming power to heal itself.

We all suppress emotions in one way or another. It is better for your health to bring forward your anger, but it is not always socially acceptable to act out your true emotions. In one of his books, Dr. Sarno gives the example of a mother who sprinkled ice water on the face of her two-year-old son whenever he threw a temper tantrum. The child settled down and the technique curbed his anger, but it was suppressed. Ice water was a very effective method of ending the temper tantrum, but this is a classic example of where the anger becomes subconscious and will eventually try to erode the conscious mind. Dr. Sarno describes these repressed emotions as "prisoners under lock and key...always trying to escape to the surface."

When I was a child, I developed severe chest pains for several months. I had been clinically diagnosed with rheumatic heart disease, which had later been ruled out. The problem had not been in the heart. I now believe it was TMS that had targeted my chest wall muscles.

The syndrome starts in your mind, but it mainly targets your muscles, fascia and nerves. These tissues become deprived of adequate blood flow and as a result, lack appropriate levels of oxygen. This partial lack of oxygen in the nerves and muscles can be very painful. The muscles then turn into knots, which we call "trigger points."

Trigger points are local areas of severe muscle spasms. These muscles go into spasms is because that is the way muscles communicate with us. The muscles are telling us that they are not getting enough nutrients—and oxygen is a vital nutrient. The tissues cannot live without oxygen, and they become sore to the touch. For example, when a person dies, the muscles stop getting oxygen and as result, the muscles go into severe, generalized spasms, which we call "rigor mortis." Rigor mortis tells us that the muscles lack nutrition.

Dr. Sarno's fascinating books made a lot of sense to me. I felt as if I were in every paragraph and sentence of his books. I had all the signs and symptoms, and my history matched perfectly with what he described as TMS. Dr. Sarno described the location and pattern of pain and it matched my symptoms exactly. The location of the trigger points are at the top of the shoulders, in the trapezius muscles, at the junction where the second ribs meet the sternum, in the muscles along the spinal column, in the outer gluteus muscles and in the outer thighs (called the IT band). I was a classic case of a person with TMS.

He also described the people who develop this syndrome as having certain personality traits. They are conscientious, hard-working, competitive perfectionists. They strive to do acts of kindness and they place everyone else's interests above their own—personality traits that I definitely had. I could never say "no" to anyone during my practice, which is often typical for people who develop TMS.

I began to think back to when my pain had started, in an attempt to analyze the onset of the whole disease process. I found out that my neck abnormality could be normal happenstance for a fifty-nine-year-old person. It was a normal part of aging—spinal compressions and other degenerative diseases happen as we age.

Dr. Sarno believes that in most cases, spinal stenosis does not need surgical correction. He believes that these are degenerative spine problems—something he calls the "gray hair of the spine." I should have realized that something similar was affecting my hands as well, as they were the most used and active muscles in my body. I didn't realize that they were telling me that they weren't getting enough of something vital. If I had known from the beginning what I know now, I would never have consented to my surgery.

Don't ever think that the x-ray diagnosis of your back condition is the final conclusion. Just because an MRI shows an abnormality does not mean that it is linked to the problem or to your symptoms. If it becomes clear that you do in fact need surgery, look for minimally invasive surgeries that are less risky and in some cases more successful. Before you jump into anything or spend thousands of dollars on medical bills and prescription drugs, first look at your personal life. Look for areas of stress or aggravation.

My retirement had been the death of something that I'd loved so dearly. My career had been my life. And the trauma that my early retirement caused had created a lot of anger and rage. I'd pushed all the horrible emotions of loss and regret deep inside of me and never let myself grieve. Retirement had placed even more tension on my condition.

During my three years of retirement, almost every

night, I dreamt that I was treating patients and operating on people. And after my own extended research, I believe that my repressed emotions about my early retirement caused the myofascial disorders, or TMS by Dr. Sarno's definition.

The Endemic

After I read all of Dr. Sarno's books, I realized that my original problem was definitely tension myositis syndrome and not spinal stenosis. Unfortunately, in today's medicine, doctors do not recognize that diagnosis and a majority of physicians do not even know what TMS is.

I called Dr. Sarno and talked to him about my case. We decided that my symptoms were a severe case of TMS. Years of surgical training and working as a practicing surgeon had created rage inside of me. I was consistently ignoring myself as a person, and that by itself caused the anger.

Back pain and myofascial disorders are common among highly civilized countries. They are quite rare in primitive societies. In the Western societies, back pain has even reached epidemic levels, with about eighty percent of all people developing back pain at some point in their lifetimes.

The most significant factor in the treatment of TMS is total belief in the diagnosis. You need to believe in it so much that you could throw out any other diagnosis. If you have a hard time accepting the diagnosis of TMS and continue to cling to an old diagnosis, your health will not get better. You must throw out the structural diagnosis. Most of the time, the diagnosis is not the cause of the symptoms.

Unfortunately, most of us are brainwashed by MRI findings and structural diagnoses that offer quick surgical fixes. Back pain is a complex problem. We need to realize that the mind plays a huge role in chronic pain.

You see, we know that the brain has total control over the blood supply of the muscle and nerves through the autonomic nervous system. The autonomic nervous system is part of the peripheral nervous system, which controls the involuntary functions of the body such as the heart rate, respiration and the movements of the muscles of the bowels. It is the same mechanism that makes your face blush when you are embarrassed or makes you look pale when you are scared.

We do not have any control over this system. Therefore, the autonomic nervous system can also make you experience oxygen deprivation by selectively cutting down the circulation to the muscles and nerves. Oxygen deficit can be very painful to the tissues. It can cause muscles to go into spasms and form painful knots.

I believe that the autonomic nervous system also plays a similar role in the development of peptic ulcer disease (stomach and duodenal ulcers). It increases the total output of acid, which has some effect on producing the ulcer. In the case of irritable bowel syndrome, the tension also has an effect through the autonomic nervous system, creating symptoms in the bowels.

Operating on different areas of the human body over the years, I'd noticed that a network of small capillaries surround the nerves—their source of blood supply. The brain has complete control over this network of capillaries. It can make them constricted and small, with diminished blood flow. The result is oxygen deprivation. The tissues that are oxygen deprived are more acidic and produce more lactic acid than normal tissues. This acidic media can irritate the nerve ending, causing pain. It is important to note that this is only one reason for oxygen deprivation, as the process is much more complex.

twelve

Living With TMS

Enlightening as Dr. Sarno's book was, as a Western-trained physician, it was hard for me to accept this diagnosis. Whenever I questioned the diagnosis in my mind, the pain level got more intense. Generally, my own fear and negative emotions created more pain. And when I thought positively, the emotion relieved the pain. This realization forced me to pay more attention to my emotions and how they affected my level of pain.

One evening, my wife and I went out with a delightful couple for dinner. The restaurant was beautiful and the company was wonderful. After I came home, I noticed that my pain level was much less than it had been before dinner. The significance of human bonding, social interaction and positive emotions on the treatment of chronic pain is immense.

Another evening, when I was at home, I was in a lot of pain. The weather was terrible, and suddenly, a bolt lightning hit a portion of the house. My wife and I had to call the fire department to advise them of the damage. Waiting for them to come, I began pacing from one end of the house to the other with practically no pain. It was amazing, but my muscles were not stiff and I could walk easily. Even after the problem was over, I felt better for a couple of hours.

I wondered what had caused this painless episode, because obviously, I had not had time to pay attention to my back during those critical moments. It was strange. When I had been doing procedures at the office, I could stand on my feet for hours with no pain, but now, I could not stand for five minutes to shave. When I'd been doing procedures, I'd been unaware of the pain.

While monitoring my pain level, I read Dr. Sarno's books over and over, and noticed significant pain reduction in my back and legs. The change was more drastic if I genuinely believed in what he said. But sometimes, due to my years of training in Western medicine, it was difficult to blindly accept his theory. If what Dr. Sarno said was true and the muscles and nerves were deprived of adequate oxygen, then increasing blood flow to those tissues, at least on temporary basis, should help the pain.

The first thing that came to mind was to do aerobic exercises, to pump more blood into my deprived muscles and nerves. I did exercises to increase my heart rate, and I saw a decrease in my pain level afterwards. Because I could not exert the muscles below my waist, I had to work on my upper body or walk on a treadmill. The other method was the application of heat and taking hot baths, which, again, helped only for a brief time.

Sleep was another key aspect to my health. People with chronic pain do not get enough quality sleep. The sleep is interrupted, which does not allow for very important REM sleep. The characteristics of REM sleep are rapid eye movement, rapid respiration and paralysis of voluntary muscles. This is the period of time when the body repairs itself through secretion of a growth hormone. Interestingly enough, there has been a study done on healthy volunteers who were deprived of REM sleep, and in four days, they all developed myofascial pain.

Lack of sleep makes muscular pain much worse. We all need about eight hours of good, quality sleep. Even those of us without chronic pain fail to get the good, quality sleep as we did over a hundred years ago.

I tried a number of natural and prescription medications to increase my REM sleep, which helped greatly. If you are looking to try this, make sure you choose short-acting medications, so that when you wake up in the morning you feel refreshed and not drowsy. These medications can be natural, herbal medications or prescription items that can be prescribed by your physician.

Taking melatonin—up to three milligrams, about two to three hours before sleep—can help. This is a natural hormone that is produced by the pineal gland in the base of the brain. It is also a great antioxidant and protects our DNA. The production of melatonin is inhibited by light and permitted in the dark, so it is produced at night, when the lights are off. People who work night shifts and sleep during the day have a much lower levels of melatonin.

Another great natural enhancer is kava kava. Taking one to three 250-milligram capsules at night can be very beneficial for both sleep and pain. It is an extract taken from the root of the kava plant, usually grown in loose, well-drained soil in the Pacific islands.

From 200 to 400 milligrams of 5 HTP (5 hydroxytryptophan) is also a safe option. This is an amino acid that will convert to the neurotransmitter hormone tryptophan—"the happy hormone." There are also prescription drugs that are short-acting and effective in creating eight hours of good sleep. These are Ambien, Lunesta, Desyrel, Klonopin and Zanaflex.

It is important to realize that it takes a few months for you to feel the difference in your body from a good night's sleep. Additionally, I made sure I did not watch the news or a movie before I went to bed because they could be full of negative things that would keep me from sleeping well.

I also began taking a Myers cocktail—a natural medication given intravenously. It is usually a combination of five to ten grams of vitamin C, combined with vitamins B1, B6, B5 and B12, and about two grams of magnesium sulfate or chloride. It is given in an IV (250 ml) of a half of normal saline or distilled water in an hour. I had that every week for eight weeks before I slowed it down to every month.

Magnesium dilates the blood vessels and increases the blood flow to the muscles. About eighty percent of Americans are deficient in magnesium because of our diet. The latest government studies revealed that about seventy percent of Americans do not consume the recommended daily intake of magnesium. If you visit the National Institute of Health Website about magnesium, it says that magnesium is needed for more than 300 biochemical reactions in the body. The usual blood tests do not reflect the magnesium deficiency and they are not accurate.

Magnesium is an intracellular element and it may be better to measure the amount in the red blood cells.

As a good as magnesium is, I do not think it reverses what the brain is doing to the blood vessels in myofascial disorders or TMS. But, in my case, it helped me, at least on a temporary basis. I learned that even if one gets pain relief on a temporary basis, it is important because you can hang on to that experience for a while and keep that in your cell memory.

Besides magnesium, I have also seen people with chronic pain respond to extra doses of B vitamins, such as B1, B6 and B12. People who are under constant stress require a large amount of B vitamins. Vitamin C is also a very good antioxidant, anti-inflammatory agent, and I have found it to be very effective for pain relief.

It's important to get a hormonal evaluation. The amount of hormones—the growth hormone, testosterone, thyroid and DHEA—in my blood were very low for a man my age. People with chronic pain frequently have a low level of growth hormone and testosterone.

I consulted physicians specialized in this field and got replacements for some of these hormones. The hormones increased my sense of wellbeing and my energy, and generally made me feel good. They also increased my self-confidence, my lean body mass and my bone density. While you take replacement hormones, you have to be monitored on regular basis—which is what I did for myself.

Another thing that seems to work for many people is guided imagery. Guided imagery is a powerful and effective healing method. You direct your thoughts to positive and constructive events. You have to visualize pleasant things that you like to do. After repeated exposure to these thoughts, the body adapts itself to parallel the thought process. I began to imagine that I was playing racquetball, envisioning all the details of the court, the ball and even the sweaty smell. Our thoughts and emotions can affect our health because our mind and body are not separated from each other. They function as a whole unit.

Each one of us is made up of a vibrant system with strong self-healing abilities. I had to remind myself that despite the fact that the spinal surgery had distorted my spinal anatomy by fusion, my body could still restore itself.

As a surgeon, I witnessed what the body can do to restore itself. I had once done a vasectomy on a patient. I'd removed about two centimeters of his vas deferens from each side, tied the ends and put them as far away from each other as possible. Five years later, the ends had actually connected back to each other, which had caused his wife to get pregnant. And I'd gotten sued because of the body's natural ability to go back to normal.

Sometimes, if we block out negative imagery of poor

health, we can actually become healthier. Although it may be difficult, we should not allow negative pictures to appear in our minds. Unfortunately, I learned this the hard way by having negative discussions about my back with the spine surgeon. The conversation had always been about how deteriorated and compressed my spine was, and those images had totally destroyed my confidence. Immediately, I would feel my pain level rise. This had been guided imagery in a negative way. If I'd had positive conversations with my doctor, maybe the pain would not have always been so excruciating.

This concept of pain in the mind goes as far back as ancient Egypt and Greece. Aristotle and Hippocrates considered that a long-standing image of a disease could eventually create its symptoms. I am not alluding to the fact that we should rule out or dismiss x-ray findings, or never take an MRI. While we should be honest and discuss the evidence, we should also say that these facts may be normal findings for a person's age and physiology, and not rush to surgery.

We all have bodies that age, and it is natural that we want to fix every twitch and spasm, but it is not always wise to actually do so. In my case, it wasn't. The surgery fixed the deformity and spinal stenosis in my back, but it took away five years of my life.

Coming to terms with my real problem—TMS—is something that I am managing successfully. However, I also have to manage the other problems that surgery created for me. I feel as though these things could have simply been prevented if I had been looked at as a patient and not as an x-ray.

thirteen

The Mind-body Connection

What we think is what we are and become. We become the products of our thought process.

—*Buddha*

After five years of suffering from my own chronic pain, I became convinced that chronic illness in general has a common cause: The mind's great influence on how we feel. Our thoughts create a certain biochemistry that invites and, in fact, hosts chronic illness.

When I looked at this concept, I thought of my years of surgery and treating cancer patients. Most of them had dealt with chronic rage and anger for years before cancer could find homes in their bodies. They could not forget nor forgive the conflicts they had endured for years. It is my belief that this rage, anger and resentment produce dreadful chemicals in the body that create an environment for chronic illness to dwell. In the case of cancer, these chemicals will destroy the immune system. Disease has to do with how much negativity and pessimism you feel over your lifetime.

Scientific research on mind-body interaction supports the fact that optimism and laughter are integral parts of the healing process. Optimism produces healthy biochemicals in our bodies, which create an environment in which it is *unsuitable* for illnesses to harbor. Chronic illnesses cannot grow in well-balanced, emotional bodies, just as bacteria cannot grow in a medium that has antibiotics in it. Happy thoughts, laughter, strong faith, love and gratitude are all positive emotions that eliminate chronic illness.

The Power of Positive Thinking

Another great book that moved me was the *Anatomy of an Illness* by Norman Cousins. He had developed a fatal condition called ankylosing spondylitis, which is an autoimmune disease that affects the connective tissues of the joints. He had been told that the chances of recovery for him were one in 500. He had been aware of the effect of negative emotion on the body and he'd thought his condition had been caused by negative emotions he had been subjected to.

If that had been the factor causing the disease, he asked himself, what could positive emotion have done for it? Could positive emotion, like laughter, love, a strong will to live and gratitude, create a chemical factor that helps cure the condition?

Cousins dedicated himself to producing positive emotions for several months. He watched the Marx Brothers movies and *Candid Camera* reruns, and consumed large doses of vitamin C through an IV. Soon, he cured his illness permanently.

He found that positive emotions created a biochemical environment that could cure some illnesses. It was a testament to the unlimited potential of the human mind. I believe that all diseases start with negative thoughts and that love, gratitude and laughter are the most potent healers.

Unfortunately, conventional medicine has the attitude that if something cannot be verified in the lab, it is considered unscientific and therefore unprovable. So, how can you demonstrate and verify the effect of emotion in a lab experience? The task is every difficult.

Fear Is the Crucial Cause

The seed of fear usually becomes implanted in someone's mind as soon as an abnormal MRI surfaces. I am specifically talking about MRI findings that happen to be very common in the normal population and do not cause any particular symptoms. Yes, the patient may have some symptoms of back and leg pain. But most of the time, the MRI findings are not the real cause of pain.

Physicians blame the structural abnormalities they see to be the cause of the symptoms. They were trained that way. They simply tell you that based on your MRI, your spine is degenerated, or that you have a disc that is causing your pain. Negative words cause fear. If you cannot see what the mind is doing to the body, then you begin to blame the symptoms on your previous medical records and MRI findings.

You become fearful of everything after you become aware of your abnormal x-ray findings. You fear physical exercise—fearing that you will injure your back further by moving the wrong way or putting too much strain on it. You begin to walk around tense all the time, afraid that the deterioration in your spine might progress into something worse. And that alone can make the pain much worse, limiting your activities.

> Fear makes cowards of us; it makes us to
> do things we should not do and keeps us
> afraid to do things we should.
>
> —Venice Bloodworth

I am not suggesting that you ignore all the findings of your MRI, no matter what your symptoms are. These are important tests and part of the armamentarium of work-up for chronic back pain. However, the findings need to be more carefully evaluated by your physician. The test results are *part* of the equation, not the solution. A patient has to be totally evaluated before a diagnosis can be made. Paying attention to the comprehensive history and progress of the patient with other alternative treatments is in the patient's best interest. Doctors need to perform a total patient evaluation of the body, mind and spirit before determining a diagnosis.

I believe that the cause of such high numbers of people with back pain is not structural abnormalities. Instead, as Dr. Sarno mentions, the cause is internal rage, anger and tension that have accumulated over the years. I saw the rage in the faces of the people who waited hours at pain clinics. It was not clear if the rage was due to the chronic pain or if it was pre-existing rage that caused the chronic pain. The mind-body interconnection was completely bombarded with negativity, and the doctors and therapists all found other physical things in the body to blame the pain on.

Unfortunately, we do not yet have any tests that can clearly see the chemistry of the body. All we have are the MRI and associated physical tests. It would be revolutionary if we could identify that bad molecule or peptide causing the pain. But we are just not that advanced—or are we?

My behavior changed twenty years ago, after I had a CAT scan done on my spine. It showed a curvature and degeneration, and that became deeply ingrained in my mind. Suddenly, I pegged myself as having a problem, even though I showed no symptoms. But the abnormality was there, haunting me all the time. Looking back, it seems crazy that I was so worried about a deformity that caused no symptoms. I wish someone could have pointed it out to me back then.

fourteen

Replacing Negative Thoughts With Positive Ones

Back pain is one of the most common sources of disability in civilized, Western societies. It is also the second most frequent pain people experience, the first being headaches.

Chronic pain syndrome has become an epidemic in this country. The problem is that we do not know how to treat chronic illness, and unfortunately, it is also the major cause of economic loss to the people it affects.

American medicine is among the best in the world when it comes to taking care of acute illnesses. But somehow, that gives us the mindset that we are able to do the same thing for chronic illnesses. This is not only untrue, but it offers false confidence. Most chronic illnesses develop over many years and are the direct result of negative mind-body interaction. You cannot ignore this proven influence of the mind over the body. The mind is not separate from the body, but what holds it all together. In Western medicine, doctors and students know little about this influence of the mind on the body, and many disregard it.

Fortunately, in the last twenty years, some medical professionals have come to the conclusion that the mind-body interaction is an affective means of the treatment of coronary artery diseases. An article was written in the *Journal of Cardiopulmonary Rehabilitation* in 1999 (Rutledge JC, Hyson DA, Garduno D, et al.) called, "Lifestyle modification program in management of patients with coronary artery disease: The clinical experience in a tertiary care hospital" (19(4):226-234).

Negative emotions can weaken and destroy the immune system. A lot of people have probably experienced this when they were under a lot of stress. They tended to develop a cold, the flu or cold sores, which are all caused by the activation of and overcoming of a virus by the immune system. I also learned in the practice of surgery that patients who had a positive outlook had fewer complications and healed faster. Unfortunately, they do not teach this information in any surgical residency program and there is no mention of it in any surgical textbooks. In my opinion, there should be a chapter devoted to the effects of emotions on the post-operative outcome.

This effect also applies to back pain. Negative emotions, such as stress, anger, rage and hopelessness, can increase the incidence and severity of pain. And, often, it is impossible to get rid of pain without eliminating those negative emotions first. This has been scientifically demonstrated in several clinical trials wherein positive mind-body interaction reduced the amount and severity of pain.

A comprehensive review called Alternative Therapies in Health and Medicine was conducted by Stanford University on mind-body therapies in the treatment of musculoskeletal disorders in the elderly. Practitioners and researchers looked into the effects of community support, cognitive-behavioral therapy, meditation, the placebo effect, imagery, visualization, spiritual/energy healing, music therapy, hypnosis, yoga, tai chi and qigong. All of these techniques were found to be effective, first and foremost, as complementary treatments for musculoskeletal disease and its associated disorders.

As for my condition, I learned that the best way to get rid of negative emotions is to immediately replace them with positive ones. If you let negativity consume your thoughts, it will proliferate and become larger and larger. And in the end, it will become gigantic and hard to handle.

A set of x-ray findings may show degeneration, stenosis, malalignment, herniated disks and similar things. True as they may be, they are all negative. Unfortunately, Western medicine has only one tool to treat these kinds of illnesses: surgery. Like Bernard Baruch said, "If all you have is a hammer, everything else looks like a nail."

2008

I currently have a structural abnormality in my back. It is called spodylolisthesis between the L4-5 vertebrae, which is a misalignment between these two vertebrae, with one in front of the other. I did not have this condition before my surgery, but Western doctors insisted that all the pain I'd had could be attributed to this specific abnormality. The treatment they had offered had been more fusions and more surgery. And what would have come after that, only God can predict.

Making the decision to rebut this diagnosis was the healthiest thing I could have done for myself. My own therapy and research was the only reason I was able to go back to my normal activities—my normal life.

In the future, back pain must be treated differently. However, the mind-body connection will not be initially beneficial to patients suffering from:

- Structural abnormality of the spines with bladder and bowel problems.
- Structural abnormalities that progress toward severe weakness and paralysis.
- Structural abnormalities that do not respond to alternative therapy including attention to a person's mid-body interaction.
- Trauma to the spine with unstable vertebrae, which need to be fused and stabilized.

fifteen

How You Can Do Things Differently

I know what you're thinking: If a trained surgeon can be subjected to several unnecessary surgeries, the rest of us don't stand a chance. That's exactly why I am writing this book. You do have a chance. You just have to start questioning doctors and looking for alternatives to spinal surgery.

First of all, I think it's important to mention some definite distinctions in pain and corrective surgery. There is no question that spinal surgery must be performed for spinal fractures that can make the spine incredibly unstable. Spinal surgery for severe congenital deformities is also justifiably indicated. And, there is little question about the need for spinal surgery for the people who have spinal stenosis and compression combined with bladder and bowel incontinence.

Otherwise, if you have degenerative spine disease like I had, with none of the above conditions, I suggest you ask an abundance of questions before you succumb to any form of surgery. You need to ask about the outcome of these surgeries for the degenerative disease. But don't expect to get clear-cut answers—I never did. Spine surgeons do not have all the answers. Back pain and myofascial disorders are very complex. And to be completely honest, I was scared to death. I was constantly thinking about paralysis, and anything looked better than that.

Major spinal surgery should be the last resort, if it's performed at all. It is my belief that ninety percent of the time, the cause of back pain has nothing to do with what is seen on your MRI. Start demanding more from your doctor, especially when surgery is a possibility.

What You Should Do

Here are some things you should think about if you have chronic back pain:

- An operation will not help when you suffer from deep-seated anger and depression. The pain will go away when you find peace within yourself.
- Chronic back pain is usually a complex problem. An MRI does not tell the entire story because it only looks at one dimension.
- Take a look at your whole life. The past, the present and the future. The worries, stress, depression, anger and resentment or recent episodes of pressures in life. Are you a person who can never say "NO" to anyone in your life? Are you the type to ignore your interests and place the welfare of everyone else on the top? Are you a "good person"? The one who wants to please 100 percent of the people 100% percent of the time? Are you a person who avoids confrontation and keeps everything inside? Are you a chronic worrier? Are you a perfectionist? Do you kick yourself all

the time? And are you your own worst critic?
- Does your pain variable change with different emotional situations around you?
- Does your pain move from one side to another? Is it better when you exercise? Is it worse at night, when you sleep?
- Are you having other symptoms beside back pain, like symptoms of irritable bowl syndrome, migraine headache, ulcer symptoms, neck pain, chest wall pain not related to your heart, or frequent urination?

If the answers to the last few questions are "yes," then be very careful that you do not let anyone operate on your back until you have analyzed all of these situations. If you have an operation for something that is not the cause of your pain, you are going to make the situation even more complicated and confusing. The pain will not go away, or it may go away temporarily and eventually come back with more intensity. Then, the issue will worsen.

No one will tell you that you didn't need the operation in the first place. Your pain will be blamed on a number of things that are mostly structural in nature. Either you'll be told that you have developed scar tissue in that area or that you have another sort of abnormality that needs to be fixed with additional surgery.

At this point, your condition will probably be called failed back syndrome, which is a basket-case diagnosis. It is not your back that failed—it was the doctor's diagnosis that failed. Don't let five years of your precious life be wasted on going from one clinic to another. Your life doesn't have to be placed on hold. Pain causes more pain, anxiety causes more anxiety and frustration causes a spiraling pit of despair.

This is not only my story, but anecdotal information from many, many people from the pain clinics, physical therapy clinics, chat rooms and minimally invasive spinal surgery centers. These people are the lost souls. They lost their spirits, and some even lost their families, because of chronic pain. They certainly lost fortunes trying to buy and purchase pain-free lives. And it all happened because of a misdiagnosis.

Doctors who practice conventional medicine do not put any emphasis on the human psyche and certainly do not want to believe that the mind may have something to do with the back—because, essentially, treating chronic back pain has become the largest industry in this country.

To the Medical Community

I am not in a position to educate my colleagues. As a matter of fact, it is inappropriate for me to do such a thing. These are my personal beliefs, based on my experiences as a patient suffering for several years after spinal surgery. Before we jump to the most aggressive treatment—surgery—patients deserve to have other areas of their lives investigated.

I would recommend that all healthcare professionals taking care of patients with chronic back pain educate themselves with Dr. Sarno's highly respected books. It was a valuable learning experience for me and his message needs to be passed on to other doctors. Dr. Sarno has had experience with more than 30,000 patients. You cannot argue with his theory because of the number of patients he has treated successfully. Physicians don't have to read only prestigious medical journals. They *must* feel obligated to examine other sources of information.

I also have a problem with the protocol of conventional medicine for the diagnosis and treatment of back pain. If the pain does not go away, almost everyone is sent for an MRI. As soon as the MRI shows some positive findings that can explain the pain, those findings overshadow everything else. At that point, the patient is referred for physical therapy, cortisone epidural injection and, if the pain does not get any better, to spine surgeons for definitive treatment of MRI abnormalities—not the definitive treatment of the patients' problems.

The conventional treatment for back pain usually does not work. Injections hardly ever work and studies prove that surgery is only effective in a small number of patients. We have to develop a different system for these cases. The patient's life should be evaluated first. They have to know what kind of person they are, where they have been, where they come from and where they are planning to go. Is this pain a manifestation and image of their personal life? Is it built-up emotional baggage from a bad relationship or childhood that has now overflowed from their mind into their muscles and found a new place to poison? This may sound crazy to the conventional medical professional, but every evolution in medicine may have sounded crazy at its foundation.

My story is about someone who had to fight drastically for many years just to get back to normalcy. The positive side of all of this is that I learned a lot from this thing called "back pain." I learned how medicine is truly practiced these days. Even though I practiced medicine for thirty years, I had no idea what damage we as physicians were causing. It was as if I was in the middle of a stream but did not know it. I could not see the forest through the trees. And then, when I saw the forest, I was shocked and completely disappointed. I learned that the practice of medicine in this country is heavily influenced by insurance companies and big industries that make medical equipment and drugs.

I also learned how the payment system for physician services varies so widely between different specialties. And, treatment options often point patients toward special procedures, like spinal surgery and spinal injections, that are lucrative for surgeons to perform. These procedures are done by a number of pain management professionals and spine surgeons. Medicare and insurance pay doctors handsomely for spinal surgery procedures and spinal injections while cardiac and vascular surgeons, who perform lifesaving procedures, get almost nothing.

I am not saying that physicians operate only for economic rewards, as that is certainly not the case. What I am saying is that we are all humans and tend to believe in things that will mostly benefit us.

I want to leave you with a quote that is a truism in today's medical world:

> Disease and ill health are caused largely by damage at the molecular and cellular level, yet today's surgical tools are too large to deal with that kind of problem.
>
> —Ralph Merkle

sources

1 Dr. John E. Sarno's books include: *Healing Back Pain: The Mind-Body Connection*, *The Divided Mind: The Epidemic of Mindbody Disorders*, *The Mindbody Prescription: Healing the Body, Healing the Pain* and *Mind Over Back Pain.*